Annual Review of Eating Disorders Part 2 – 2008

Edited by

Stephen Wonderlich
James E Mitchell
Martina de Zwaan
Howard Steiger

Foreword by

Kelly L Klump

RADCLIFFE PUBLISHING
OXFORD • NEW YORK

Radcliffe Publishing Ltd
18 Marcham Road
Abingdon
Oxon OX14 1AA
United Kingdom

www.radcliffe-oxford.com
Electronic catalogue and worldwide online ordering facility.

British Library Cataloguing in Publication Data

A catalogue record for this book is available from the British Library.

ISBN 978 1 84619 244 9

Typeset by Advance Typesetting Ltd, Oxford
Printed and bound by TJ International Ltd, Padstow, Cornwall

Contents

Foreword

As 2007–2008 President of the Academy for Eating Disorders (AED), I am pleased to provide the opening comments for the *Annual Review of Eating Disorders, Part 2, 2008*. This edition is fourth in a series of *Annual Reviews*. The AED is proud to sponsor the series, as we are the largest international organization of eating disorder professionals in the world. Our membership is multidisciplinary and global, reflecting the range of professionals needed to combat eating disorders and all of their complexity. Our members are leading experts in the research, treatment, and prevention of eating disorders. We are thankful for the opportunity to showcase their work in the *Annual Review*.

Much like previous *Annual Reviews*, this edition includes an impressive collection of comprehensive reviews covering the state-of-the-science in the eating disorders field. These reviews evaluate clinical and empirical data published in 2004–2006 examining issues as diverse as neurobiological influences, body image, and treatment of eating disorders. The depth and scope of the reviews are a testament to the hard work of the editors and the authors who volunteered their time for this important project. We are grateful for their contributions and look forward to continued collaborations on future editions of the *Annual Review*.

Kelly L Klump PhD
President, Academy for Eating Disorders
August 2007

List of editors

Stephen Wonderlich PhD
Professor and Associate Chair, Neuropsychiatric Research Institute and Department of Clinical Neuroscience, University of North Dakota School of Medicine and Health Sciences, Fargo, North Dakota, USA

James E Mitchell MD
Professor and Chairman, Neuropsychiatric Research Institute and Department of Clinical Neuroscience, University of North Dakota School of Medicine and Health Sciences, Fargo, North Dakota, USA

Martina de Zwaan MD
Professor of Psychosomatic Medicine and Psychotherapy, University of Erlangen-Nuremberg, Erlangen, Germany

Howard Steiger PhD
Director, Eating Disorders Program, Douglas Mental Health University Institute; Professor, Psychiatry Department, McGill University, Montreal, Canada

List of contributors

Evelyn Attia MD
Department of Psychiatry, Columbia University, New York, USA

Katie Bannon BA
Department of Psychology, Rutgers University, New Brunswick, USA

Amanda Joelle Brown BA
New York State Psychiatric Institute, New York, USA

Kristen M Culbert MA
Department of Psychology, Michigan State University, East Lansing, USA

Janine DesForges MB BS, BSc, MRCPsych
Mental Health Unit, Northwick Park Hospital, London, UK

Angela Favaro MD, PhD, MSc
Psychiatric Clinic, Department of Neurosciences, University of Padua, Padua, Italy

Julie A Gravener BA
Department of Psychology, University of Iowa, Iowa City, USA

Brooke E Heinicke DPsychHlthPsych
School of Psychological Science, La Trobe University, Melbourne, Victoria, Australia

Hans W Hoek MD, PhD
Parnassia Psychiatric Institute, The Hague, The Netherlands; Department of Epidemiology, Columbia University, New York, USA; Department of Psychiatry, University Medical Center, Groningen, The Netherlands

Pamela K Keel PhD
Department of Psychology, University of Iowa, Iowa City, USA

Anna Keski-Rahkonen MD, PhD, MPH
Department of Public Health, University of Helsinki, Helsinki, Finland

Kelly L Klump PhD, FAED
Department of Psychology, Michigan State University, East Lansing, USA

Bryan Lask FRCPsych MB BS, MPhil, FRCPH, FAED
Regional Eating Disorder Service, Ulleval University Hospital, Oslo, Norway; The Huntercombe Hospitals, UK; St George's University of London, UK

Mario Maj MD
Department of Psychiatry, University of Naples SUN, Naples, Italy

Palmiero Monteleone MD
Department of Psychiatry, University of Naples SUN, Naples, Italy

Maria Øverås CandPsychol
Regional Eating Disorder Service, Ulleval University Hospital, Oslo, Norway

Susan J Paxton MPsych PhD
School of Psychological Science, La Trobe University, Melbourne, Victoria, Australia

Kathleen Pike PhD
Department of Psychiatry, Columbia University, New York, USA

Anu Raevuori MD
Department of Public Health, University of Helsinki, Helsinki, Finland

Paolo Santonastaso MD
Psychiatric Clinic, Department of Neurosciences, University of Padua, Padua, Italy

Jennifer D Slane MA
Department of Psychology, Michigan State University, East Lansing, USA

Janet Treasure MD, PhD, FRCP, FRCPsych
Eating Disorders Unit, Department of Academic Psychiatry, Guy's Hospital, King's College London, UK

Kristin M von Ranson PhD
Department of Psychology, University of Calgary, Alberta, Canada

G Terence Wilson PhD
Department of Psychology, Rutgers University, New Brunswick, USA

Eirin Winje CandPsychol
Regional Eating Disorder Service, Ulleval University Hospital, Oslo, Norway

Acknowledgements

We have appreciated the opportunity to serve as Editors of the first four editions of the *Annual Review of Eating Disorders*. With these four editions we have completed one full 'cycle' in which each of the 20 eating disorder topics was reviewed over two separate time intervals. Our original intent was to provide up-to-date longitudinal critiques and reviews of these topics. We hope that the information in the *Annual Reviews* so far has been helpful to the members of the Academy and the greater eating disorder research and clinical communities.

We would like to thank the Board of Directors of the Academy for their support of this project, as well as the members of the Publication Council who helped to inform and launch the original project. We also appreciate the support of The Sherwood Group, particularly Sally Finney, who has been most supportive and helpful. Finally, we wish to thank our colleagues who graciously volunteered their knowledge and time by contributing chapters to the Reviews. We wish the Academy well in their future efforts to provide our membership with concise, clinically oriented reviews.

Finally, on a personal note we would each like to thank the following people:

Steve Wonderlich – Karen, Sara, Anna and Joe
James Mitchell – Karen, James and Katherine
Martina de Zwaan – Gisa and Sissi
Howard Steiger – Mimi, Ethel and Morris

1

Psychobiology of eating disorders

Angela Favaro, Palmiero Monteleone, Paolo Santonastaso and Mario Maj

Abstract

Objectives of review. The goal of this review is to highlight advances in research on the psychobiology of eating disorders during the period 2005–2006.

Summary of recent findings. Studies on the function of neurotransmitters such as serotonin and dopamine in eating disorders have demonstrated the presence of state- and trait-related alterations and their associations with behavioral and comorbid characteristics. Neuroendocrinological alterations that are present in anorexia nervosa (AN) appear to have significant influences on body composition, resumption of menses, and risk of developing osteoporosis. Studies of gastrointestinal peptides and adipokines have shown an association between the circulating levels of these peptides and alterations in food intake, satiety and motor activity in AN, bulimia nervosa (BN) and binge eating disorder (BED). New areas of research cover the function of neurosteroids and brain-derived neurotrophic factor, as well as the possible role of neurodevelopment in the pathogenesis of eating disorders.

Future directions. The findings from recent studies are important, but have yet to lead to significantly improved treatments and better outcome for our patients. The aim of studies in the next decade will be to elucidate the specific neurobiological, psychological and sociocultural factors that have etiological significance in eating disorders, and to try to translate these findings into more effective treatments.

Introduction

Recent research has led to remarkable advances in the methodology and knowledge of the psychobiology of eating disorders. Researchers and clinicians now possess a great deal of information about the regulation of neurotransmitters, neuropeptides, neurohormones and also peripheral peptides that influence energy metabolism, eating behavior, cognitive functioning and mood. Interestingly, this availability of knowledge and the advances in technology are the necessary conditions which enable us to understand the connections between neurobiology and the clinical aspects of eating disorders, including diagnostic characteristics, comorbidity, outcome and etiopathogenesis. One of the aims of the recent research is to establish the role of the pathophysiology of neurobiological systems in the development and maintenance of eating disorders. The first step is to determine whether neurobiological alterations are a consequence or a potential cause of pathological eating behavior or malnutrition. Moreover, biological (and psychological) disturbances observed in eating disorders might be trait or state based. In the first case, neurobiological variants and alterations represent candidate endophenotypes of eating disorders that need to be characterized and studied with regard to their origin and distribution in the family and in the population.

The previous review (Jimerson and Wolfe 2006) focused selectively on the neurotransmitter serotonin, the adipokine leptin, and the gut-related peptide ghrelin. We decided to address these three topics by giving an update of the literature for the period 2005–2006. In addition, we included in the present review other topics that were not considered in the previous one, but which have formed the focus of intensive study in recent years.

Literature review

Serotonin

Abnormalities in serotonin (5-HT) regulation are present in eating disorders both in the acute phase of the illness and after recovery (Kaye *et al.* 2005a, 2005b). Since 5-HT plays many important roles in the brain, it is important to understand which behaviors or characteristics of our patients are influenced by these abnormalities. Several studies have been performed in an attempt to better understand the impact of 5-HT function in the etiopathogenesis, maintenance and clinical characteristics of eating disorders. In BN, for example, a decrease in 5-HT activity has been associated with impulsivity, affective instability, self-harming behavior and interpersonal insecurity (Steiger *et al.* 2001, 2004).

In this area of research, Bruce *et al.* (2006) recently found significantly reduced platelet [^{3}H]-paroxetine binding in AN patients compared with controls. Paroxetine binding was inversely related to dieting preoccupations, affective instability, social avoidance, anxiousness and compulsivity. These findings suggest that certain pathological personality traits may be associated with reduced 5-HT activity in subjects with an active eating disorder. Using the same methodology, Steiger and colleagues (2006) explored the intrafamilial correspondence of 5-HT function in BN subjects and their unaffected first-degree relatives. Paroxetine binding was significantly reduced in BN subjects and their female first-degree relatives compared with controls, even after exclusion of all the relatives with a reported psychiatric disorder. Significant within-family correlations were observed, leading to the hypothesis that some heritable trait might influence both 5-HT activity and the risk of developing BN (Steiger *et al.* 2006).

Neuroimaging studies that used ligands specific to the study of 5-HT receptor activity have given further support to the research in the field. In women with AN, Bailer and colleagues (2007) conducted a study exploring the activity of both 5-HT1A and 5-HT2A serotonin receptors. They found significantly increased activity of the 5-HT1A receptor in several brain areas, whereas cerebral blood flow and 5-HT2A receptor activity were similar to those of healthy controls. However, the activity of the 5-HT1A receptors in supragenual cingulate, frontal and parietal regions was significantly correlated with harm avoidance. In a study in recovered subjects, Bailer and colleagues (2005) found that serotonin 5-HT1A receptor binding was increased in women who had recovered from binge-eating/purging type AN. In contrast, in women who had recovered from restricting AN, serotonin 5-HT1A receptor binding was not increased, but was significantly correlated with harm avoidance. Both observations support the hypothesis of serotonin-mediated persistent neurobiological alterations in AN that seem to be linked to anxiety and affect regulation.

Mondelli and colleagues (2006) performed a preliminary study to investigate the neuroendocrine response after citalopram infusion in a small sample of AN subjects and controls. The authors found that serotonergic control of anterior pituitary function, at least via the pathways activated by citalopram, was preserved in anorexia. They also observed that cortisol levels were higher following citalopram than following placebo in healthy women, but not in AN cases, thus indicating a lack of cortisol response to citalopram-induced adrenocortico-tropic hormone (ACTH) response in these patients. This finding would suggest impairment of the adrenal function.

Another approach to studying the role of 5-HT function abnormalities in AN involves the use of the 'activity-based anorexia' in animal models. Two recent studies explored the role of fenfluramine (a serotonin agonist that increases 5-HT activity) and 8-OH-DPAT (a drug that reduces serotonergic neurotransmission) in conditioning the onset and the severity of activity-based anorexia in female rats (Atchley and Eckel 2005, 2006). When fenfluramine was used, rats did not display more reduction of food intake, but did show an accelerated rate of weight loss, probably because of the effects of 5-HT on metabolism (Atchley and Eckel 2005). When 8-OH-DPAT was used, the authors observed no differences with regard to food intake, but noted a significant reduction in hyperactivity, which was linked to less severe weight loss (Atchley and Eckel 2006). In conclusion, modulation of the serotonergic system affects the development of activity-based anorexia in rats, and this lends further support to the implication of this system in the etiology of AN.

Dopamine

Animal studies show that both a dopaminergic deficit and very high levels of dopaminergic stimulation may decrease feeding (Brambilla *et al.* 2001). In addition, dopamine (DA) function seems to affect the regulation of motor activity (Casper 2006) and reward (Di Chiara 1999). The findings of previous studies of the central secretion of DA and its metabolites in AN are contradictory. In contrast, the results of pharmacological stimulation tests probing the functional state of hypothalamic postsynaptic D2 receptors and therefore, indirectly, of presynaptic DA secretion support the hypothesis of central DA hyperactivity in AN (Brambilla *et al.* 2001).

Recent studies have confirmed that DA function might have a role in eating disorders. Castro-Fornieles and colleagues (2006) found that plasma levels of homovanillic acid were significantly higher in early-onset adolescent AN subjects than in a control group of similar age. The patients with higher levels of the metabolite were those with more severe depression. In addition, improvement of weight and depression was correlated with normalization of the homovanillic acid levels. Other studies seem to suggest that abnormalities in DA function are not simply present in the acutely ill, but may be a 'trait'. Subjects with AN have an altered frequency of functional polymorphisms of the D2-receptor gene that seems to affect the efficiency of receptor transcription and translation (Bergen *et al.* 2005). A study using positron emission tomography imaging with the radioligand [^{11}C]-raclopride was performed in a sample of recovered AN subjects (Frank *et al.* 2005). The study found increased dopamine D2/D3 receptor binding, which supports the hypothesis of decreased intrasynaptic DA concentration or increased density or affinity of the D2/D3 receptors in recovered AN patients. Furthermore, the DA receptor binding was correlated with harm avoidance. According to the authors, these findings might suggest a role of DA function in some 'core' anorexic symptoms, such as eating restraint, ability to lose weight, excessive exercise, and insensitivity to normal rewards (Frank *et al.* 2005).

Hypothalamic–pituitary–adrenal (HPA) axis

Extensive evidence supports the notion of hyperactivity of the HPA axis in the acute phase of AN. Bliss and Migeon (1957) first found increased plasma levels of cortisol in underweight patients with AN. This finding was replicated by several other authors, who also reported normal circadian rhythms of cortisol and ACTH with increased plasma cortisol concentrations throughout the day, enhanced frequency and amplitude of cortisol secretory bursts, increased urinary free cortisol levels, non-suppression of cortisol after dexamethasone administration, normal or increased cortisol responses to ACTH stimulation, decreased ACTH response to corticotropin-releasing factor (CRF), and enhanced levels of CRF in the cerebrospinal fluid (CSF) (for a review, see Brambilla and Monteleone 2003). HPA axis abnormalities were shown to normalize in long-term weight-restored AN patients (for a review, see Brambilla and Monteleone 2003), and it has therefore been assumed that the HPA axis hyperactivity in underweight AN individuals is secondary to malnutrition.

Only slight modifications of HPA axis activity were reported in the acute phase of BN. Despite this, 20–60% of patients with BN were found to be non-suppressors of DST (dexamethasone suppression test) in the symptomatic phase, but not after successful treatment of BN (for a review, see Brambilla and Monteleone 2003).

In the past two years, interest has focused on exploring the role of hyper-cortisolaemia in both the determination of regional body composition and the prediction of body weight (BW) and menstrual recovery in AN. Since cortisol has antilipolytic effects, and growth hormone (GH) is lipolytic, Misra and colleagues (2005a) investigated the role of both hormones in body fat and lean mass distribution in a sample of 23 adolescents with AN. They showed that high plasma cortisol concentrations (measured as the area under the curve from 8.00 pm to 8.00 am) predicted lower lean mass in the extremities and increased lean mass in the trunk. Moreover, girls with AN who had high cortisol and low GH plasma concentrations (based on median values for both hormones in the group) were more likely to recover weight early, and their regional fat mass did not differ from that of healthy controls. Instead, girls with AN who had low cortisol and high GH levels were less likely to recover weight, and had lower trunk fat than controls. In a subsequent study by the same group (Misra *et al.* 2006a), it has been shown that girls with AN with higher cortisol levels before entering a 1-year treatment program gained more fat mass with weight gain, and their increase in body fat predicted menstrual recovery. Therefore, girls with AN who have increased cortisol concentrations seem to have a greater likelihood of menstrual recovery. The role of cortisol in predicting menstrual recovery in AN may stem not from its effect on the gonadal axis, which actually seems to be inhibitory (Saketos *et al.* 1993), but from the effect on body composition in AN (Misra *et al.* 2005a).

Finally, in a small open study that included only five women with restricting-type AN (Schule *et al.* 2006), the antidepressant mirtazapine (at a dose of 45 mg/day over three weeks) has been shown to decrease daytime salivary cortisol concentrations, with a trend towards an increase in BW, suggesting that interventions which aim to decrease HPA axis activity may be of therapeutic value in AN. Double-blind placebo-controlled studies are needed to verify this hypothesis.

As for BN, Birketvedt and colleagues (2006) observed decreased diurnal secretion of cortisol (from 6.00 am to 2.00 pm), which tended to excessively increase after daytime meals, and an enhanced ACTH response to CRF admin-istration in a small sample of female remitted BN patients. Therefore, although in remitted BN patients the adrenal glands seem to show hyposecretion of cortisol during the daytime, they show a hyperactive response to both physio-logical stimuli (meals) and exogenous CRF. Even if this study needs replication, it may suggest the persistence of dysregulation of the HPA axis in BN, which may represent a vulnerability factor for the development of eating disorders.

Hypothalamic–growth hormone–insulin-like growth factor I axis

In emaciated AN women, increased plasma levels of GH and reduced plasma concentrations of insulin-like growth factor I (IGF-I), GH binding protein (GHBP) and IGF-I binding proteins (IGFBP), especially IGFBP-3, were commonly observed (for a review, see Brambilla and Monteleone 2003). The decreases in IGF-I, GHBP and IGFBP levels point to a state of GH resistance, which is probably the reason why hypersecretion of GH in emaciated AN patients does not result in acromegalic manifestations. Both increased and normal baseline GH levels with normal circadian rhythm as well as normal or reduced circulating IGF-I were observed in individuals with BN (for a review, see Brambilla and Monteleone 2003).

From a clinical point of view, the dysregulation of the hypothalamic–GH–IGF-I axis together with hypercortisolaemia and hypoestrogenaemia could be involved in the pathogenesis of osteopenia, since IGF-I has a trophic effect on the bone, by stimulating the proliferation and differentiation of osteoblast precursors and promoting collagen synthesis. Strong correlations were reported between bone mass density (BMD) values and variables reflecting nutritional status, such as BMI, body fat, IGF-I and leptin in underweight AN patients (Grinspoon et al. 1999; Soyka et al. 2002). Data concerning osteopenia in BN are contradictory, with some studies reporting normal BMD and others reporting decreased BMD in symptomatic bulimic patients (Newton et al. 1993; Zipfel et al. 2001).

Recent studies attempted to find effective methods to correct osteopenia in underweight AN patients by administering anabolic agents to improve decreased bone formation, and to inhibit osteoclast-mediated bone resorption. Miller and colleagues (2005) randomized 33 women with AN and relative testosterone deficiency to transdermal testosterone, 150 µg or 300 µg, or placebo, for three weeks. Testosterone administration resulted in an increase in some but not all bone formation markers, together with a significant improvement in mood, spatial cognition and well-being. In a pilot study, aledronate, a potent aminobisphosphonate that inhibits bone resorption and has been proved to increase BMD and reduce fracture risk in post-menopausal women (Lieberman et al. 1995), was administered for 1 year to adolescents with AN (Golden et al. 2005). Aledronate significantly increased BMD of the lumbar spine and femoral neck, but these results were not statistically significant when compared with placebo. Further larger studies are needed to test the efficacy of this or other similar compounds in reverting osteopenia in AN.

Endocrine and nutrition-related factors that predict BMD in BN subjects were assessed in a relatively large sample of 77 women with BN compared with 56 age- and BMI-matched healthy controls (Naessén et al. 2006). BN subjects had a significantly lower spinal BMD and higher frequency of osteopenia in the total body than controls. Moreover, they showed significantly reduced levels of 17-estradiol and free thyroxine, and increased cortisol concentrations, but normal levels of testosterone, free testosterone and IGF-I. Although, in univariate analysis, a history of amenorrhea, cortisol levels, testosterone levels, previous AN and BMI were significantly associated with spinal BMD, subsequent multiple regression analysis revealed previous AN to be the strongest and only determinant of BMD. This suggests that factors which act during the AN phase may have impaired BMD, which remained decreased even after shifting to a full BN syndrome.

Gastrointestinal peptides and adipokines

The gastrointestinal tract and adipose tissue produce numerous substances and hormones that are known to have a role in the regulation of energy metabolism and eating behavior. Therefore alterations in the physiology of these substances have been supposed to occur in both AN and BN. In recent years, in patients with eating disorders, attention has focused mainly on the adipose-tissue-derived hormones leptin, adiponectin and resistin, and on the gastrointestinal peptides ghrelin and PYY.

Adiponectin

Adiponectin is a protein hormone that is produced exclusively by adipocytes and which has been shown to modulate insulin sensitivity. Decreased adiponectin production has been supposed to be involved in the development of obesity, diabetes and insulin resistance (Havel 2002). In underweight patients with AN, elevated levels of circulating adiponectin were reported by some authors (Delporte *et al.* 2003; Pannacciulli *et al.* 2003). By contrast, Iwahashi and colleagues (2003) did not observe any difference in adiponectin concentration between AN patients and healthy women, whereas Tagami and colleagues (2004) found decreased levels in malnourished individuals with AN.

During the last two years, the presence of increased levels of adiponectin in AN patients has been confirmed by three independent research groups (Bosy-Westphal *et al.* 2005; Housova *et al.* 2005; Dostalova *et al.* 2006a). Moreover, adiponectin was found to be strictly correlated with the patients' nutritional status, since an inverse correlation between hormone concentration and both BMI and percentage body fat mass was demonstrated (Housova *et al.* 2005; Dostalova *et al.* 2006a). Less severely malnourished patients with the binge/purge subtype of AN showed a relatively modest increase in circulating adiponectin levels, whereas a more prominent rise in this parameter was found in severely malnourished individuals with restrictive AN (Housova *et al.* 2005). In a sample of AN patients undergoing BW recovery, elevated pretreatment adiponectin levels only declined minimally after weight gain. This suggests that factors other than changes in body fat mass are involved in the determination of dysregulated adiponectin production in AN. The physiological relevance of high adiponectin levels in AN is unclear. Two main hypotheses have been put forward. The first one suggests that, since intracerebroventricular administration of adiponectin in mice decreases BW (Qi *et al.* 2004), hyperadiponectinemia could be a contributing etiopathogenetic factor in AN (Housova *et al.* 2005). Alternatively, elevated circulating adiponectin concentrations might represent a compensatory mechanism for the increased insulin sensitivity in patients with AN, since a negative correlation between plasma adiponectin and insulin was found in these patients (Dostalova *et al.* 2006a). In patients with BN, one study reported increased concentrations of adiponectin that showed a positive correlation with the severity of binge/purging (Monteleone *et al.* 2003), whereas another study (Tagami *et al.* 2004) detected decreased circulating levels of the adipokine. Housova and colleagues (2005) found normal concentrations of adiponectin in symptomatic bulimic women. Differences in the patients' samples, the assay methods and the time of day when blood was collected may be responsible for these discrepancies between the studies.

Resistin

Resistin has been proposed as a regulator of insulin action representing a potential link between obesity and insulin resistance (Steppan *et al.* 2001). In a study by Housova and colleagues (2005), plasma resistin levels in patients with AN were not found to be significantly different from those in controls or in patients with BN, and showed no significant relationship to BMI or body fat content. In contrast, significantly decreased plasma resistin levels were detected in AN patients by Dostalova and colleagues (2006a, 2006b), who suggested that low plasma resistin levels in AN were probably related to a defective mononuclear-macrophage number and/or function, since in humans resistin, in addition to being produced in adipocytes, is secreted in large amounts by macrophages in the bone marrow (Patel *et al.* 2003). Interestingly, in an *in vivo* microdialysis experiment, increased levels of resistin were found in the subcutaneous adipose tissue of undernourished AN patients (Dostalova *et al.* 2006b). The reasons for and significance of these opposite changes in resistin in the blood and adipose tissue of individuals with AN need to be understood.

Leptin

Leptin acts functionally as an adipocyte-derived factor that informs the central nervous system about the amount of energy stored in the body adipose tissue, and it behaves as a hunger suppressant signal involved in both the long-term and short-term regulation of energy balance (Blundell *et al.* 2001). Leptin is also a crucial hormone for many physiological processes, such as inflammation, angiogenesis, endocrine regulation, immune function and, most importantly, reproduction (Bouloumie *et al.* 1998; Fantuzzi and Faggioni 2000; Moschos *et al.* 2002).

The findings on leptin physiology in both AN and BN subjects have been comprehensively reviewed (Monteleone *et al.* 2004a; Chan and Mantzoros 2005; Jimerson and Wolfe 2006). During the last two years, researchers have further explored the secretory characteristics of the fat hormone in acutely ill malnourished anorexic patients, and after the recovery of BW, as well as its putative role in physical hyperactivity of starved individuals with AN. Circulating leptin levels and secretory characteristics were studied in adolescent girls by frequent blood sampling (every 30 minutes) overnight for 12 hours (Misra *et al.* 2005b). Low leptin levels in AN were found to be a consequence of decreased basal and pulsatile leptin secretion, and were strongly predicted by markers of nutritional status, including BMI, percentage body fat and insulin resistance index. Moreover, leptin was a predictor of GH burst frequency and burst interval, cortisol half-life and urinary free cortisol, as well as of estradiol and thyroid hormones. These data corroborate the view that, in AN, circulating leptin levels are regulated by nutritional status, and may in turn play a role in the modulation of nutritionally regulated hormones. In a study by Dostalova and colleagues (2005), in which reduced levels of leptin and increased levels of the soluble leptin receptor were found in acutely ill anorexic girls, leptin levels in the subcutaneous adipose tissue did not differ from those of healthy controls. This could mean that the nutritional changes which occur in malnourished individuals with AN do not affect leptin production by the subcutaneous adipose tissue, although they do reduce blood leptin levels. This finding was explained by the increased number of smaller adipocytes in the subcutaneous adipose tissue leading to a higher number of adipocytes per unit volume in AN subjects compared with controls. This could be responsible for the reduced efficiency of the sympathetic nervous system in inhibiting adipocyte leptin production, which would result in increased local leptin levels. On the other hand, because of the reduced volume of adipocytes, less leptin would be secreted into the circulation.

The role of leptin in the adaptation to starvation and in the process of BW recovery was investigated by two independent groups. Haas and colleagues (2005) found low leptin levels and decreased resting energy expenditure (REE) in severely malnourished women with AN. Although serum leptin levels showed a positive association with REE, this association became weaker after adjusting REE for free fat mass, and disappeared after further adjustment for serum tri-iodothyronine (T_3) concentrations. These findings prompted the authors to suggest that in starved AN patients a decrease in fat mass sensed by leptin may lead to a lowering of REE brought about by decreasing serum T_3 levels. Moreover, during weight gain, as expected, serum leptin levels increased and were associated with energy intake and REE. In particular, changes in leptin secretion occurring in the first six weeks of weight recovery were negatively associated with changes in BW between weeks six and 12 of treatment. This negative association confirms the previous suggestion that leptin should be monitored in order to slow down weight gain in AN with high leptin concentrations (Holtkamp et al. 2003), since leptin levels at discharge higher than those of healthy controls were predictive of poor outcome after one year (Holtkamp et al. 2004). In a second study, in which time-course relationships between serum leptin levels and BMI values were assessed during refeeding therapy, it was shown that BMI was significantly raised by the second week, whereas plasma leptin levels did not rise significantly up to week six of refeeding. This suggests either the existence of factors that restrict leptin production by adipocytes, or no significant change in the number of adipose cells in the first weeks of weight recovery. Either way, these findings again point to the role of leptin in the weight-gaining process.

A link between hypoleptinemia and physical hyperactivity has been shown in the animal model of semi-starvation-induced hyperactivity (Exner et al. 2000), and leptin administration has been shown to reduce this hyperactivity in rats (Hillebrand et al. 2005). Low leptin levels have been shown to correlate with hyperactivity in starved anorexic women (Hebebrand et al. 2003). It has been pointed out that activity levels were lower in severely emaciated patients with almost non-detectable leptin levels than in patients who had somewhat higher levels, which suggests that the relationship between leptin and physical activity follows an inverted U shape (Holtkamp *et al.* 2006). This finding led to the hypothesis that the postulated effect of hypolectinemia on activity levels declines when patients are close to starvation and thus critically ill, as it occurs in rats in which semi-starvation-induced hyperactivity ceases close to death (Hebebrand *et al.* 2003).

Ghrelin

Ghrelin is an endogenous 28-amino-acid peptide, initially characterized as a ligand for the growth hormone secretagogue receptor, and primarily produced by the endocrine cells in the stomach. The physiological relevance of such a localization remained unclear until it was found that this hormone plays an important role in the regulation of food intake and metabolism. In fact ghrelin is known to act as a 'hunger hormone' that signals to the brain the need to initiate food consumption (Cummings *et al.* 2001).

Fasting circulating levels of ghrelin were consistently reported to be increased in underweight patients with AN, and to normalize with the recovery of BW. In contrast, both increased and normal concentrations of the gastric hormone were found in symptomatic BN subjects (for a review, see Jimerson and Wolfe 2004, 2006). The initial claim that both AN and BN patients with binge/purging episodes had higher plasma ghrelin levels compared with non-binge/purging AN and BN patients (Tanaka *et al.* 2002, 2003a, 2003b) was not confirmed by recent larger studies (Otto *et al.* 2004; Monteleone *et al.* 2005b; Troisi *et al.* 2005). Therefore, it seems that in eating disorders, changes in the baseline secretion of ghrelin are related to nutritional status rather than to the type of abnormal eating pattern. Recently, one study reported that increased circulating levels of ghrelin in emaciated patients with restrictive AN progressively decreased during the process of BW gain to reach values even lower than those in healthy controls after three and six months of refeeding, although BMI values were still lower than the control values (Janas-Kozik *et al.* 2007). Interestingly, in this study, changes in total plasma ghrelin levels were negatively correlated with changes in BMI after 6 months of therapy. This suggests that in restrictive AN ghrelin does not send the correct information to the regulatory eating centers about the need of food consumption.

The dynamics of ghrelin secretion after energy intake have been extensively studied in emaciated AN patients, with mixed results (for a review, see Jimerson and Wolfe 2004, 2006). During the last two years evidence has been provided which suggests that the response of ghrelin to acute energy intake was almost preserved in both acutely ill and weight-recovered AN patients. Otto and colleagues (2005) showed that circulating ghrelin levels were normally decreased by a liquid meal in anorexic women either before refeeding and after partial recovery of BW, or at discharge. This suggests that in AN the suppression of ghrelin by acute changes in energy balance (feeding) was not disturbed, and was independent of chronic changes in energy balance (weight gain). Nakahara and colleagues (2007) found that circulating ghrelin secretion was increased in undernourished patients with restrictive AN, with an almost normal suppression after a test meal. After nutritional rehabilitation with partial recovery of BW, fasting plasma ghrelin levels decreased to values similar to those in normal controls, and although the response to the test meal was preserved, circulating levels were higher than the control values two and three hours after the meal, which suggests an incomplete restoration of ghrelin physiology.

One of the major issues that still need to be addressed in ghrelin research is to clarify the role of acylated (active) and desacyl (inactive) ghrelin in AN. This issue is particularly relevant because of the finding that desacyl ghrelin decreases food intake and delays gastric empting in mice and rats (Asakawa *et al.* 2005; Chen *et al.* 2005), thus showing opposite effects of the active form. Previous investigations on this topic provided conflicting results (for a review, see Jimerson and Wolfe 2006). One small study found significantly increased levels of total (acylated plus desacyl) ghrelin but slightly enhanced concentrations of the acylated ghrelin in a mixed sample of AN and BN patients (Uehara *et al.* 2005). Further studies are needed in this area.

In women with symptomatic BN, the ghrelin response to food ingestion has been reported to be consistently blunted by two independent research groups (Kojima *et al.* 2005; Monteleone *et al.* 2005b), who suggested that impaired ghrelin suppression after a meal may sustain binge eating.

Peptide YY

The short-term appetite regulator peptide YY (PYY), which belongs to the neuropeptide Y family, is a 36-amino-acid peptide secreted by the endocrine L-cells of the gut (Adrian *et al.* 1985). Circulating PYY levels are low in the fasting state and rapidly increase postprandially, when two forms, PYY_{1-36} and PYY_{3-36}, are released into the circulation (Druce *et al.* 2004). After a period of fasting, a single infusion of PYY_{3-36} is capable of reducing food intake by over a third in both lean and obese human volunteers for 24 hours, and of decreasing circulating ghrelin levels (Batterham *et al.* 2003). Therefore it appears that peripheral PYY_{3-36} acts as a satiety signal that regulates the termination of individual meals, partially by decreasing the production of the hunger-stimulating peptide ghrelin.

Studies of PYY_{3-36} secretion in people with eating disorders are still scarce. In malnourished girls with AN, baseline PYY_{3-36} levels were reported to be normal (Stock *et al.* 2005) or increased (Misra *et al.* 2006b; Nakahara *et al.* 2007), while the PYY_{3-36} response to energy intake was reported to be time-delayed (Stock *et al.* 2005) or increased (Nakahara *et al.* 2007). After partial recovery of body weight, the PYY_{3-36} response to a test meal improved, but was not completely restored (Nakahara *et al.* 2007).

With regard to BN, initial studies reported normal CSF and plasma levels of PYY in both symptomatic and one-year-recovered bulimic patients (Berrettini *et al.* 1988; Kaye *et al.* 1990). Moreover, Kaye *et al.* (1990) measured plasma concentrations of PYY in five bulimic women during episodes of binge/vomiting and in six healthy women, who experimentally binged without vomiting. In the latter, plasma PYY concentrations increased significantly after a meal and remained elevated for the next two hours. In the former, circulating PYY levels increased after the first binge and remained elevated for the duration of bingeing and vomiting. Bulimic patients had a slightly higher postprandial peak value of PYY than did healthy volunteers. Recently, two independent research groups found a blunted PYY_{3-36} response to food ingestion in symptomatic bulimic women, together with a decreased response of ghrelin (Kojima *et al.* 2005; Monteleone *et al.* 2005c). Moreover, both studies showed a negative correlation between a meal-induced increase in PPY levels and decrease in ghrelin levels, which suggests a negative interaction of PYY_{3-36} with ghrelin. The suppression of circulating ghrelin levels and the increase in plasma PYY_{3-36} levels after food ingestion may indicate the compensatory activation of peripheral signals aimed at promoting termination of food ingestion. Hence, in symptomatic bulimic patients, the blunted responses of circulating ghrelin and PYY_{3-36} levels to a test meal would indicate the occurrence in these subjects of impaired suppression of the drive to eat following a meal, which might play a role in the increased food consumption and binge eating. Further studies need to clarify the state- or trait-dependent nature of these alterations in BN.

Neurosteroids

The term 'neurosteroids' has been applied to steroid hormones such as allopregnanolone, dehydroepiendrosterone (DHEA) and its sulphated metabolite (DHEA-S), which are synthesized in the brain either *de novo* from cholesterol or by the *in situ* metabolism of bloodborne precursors (Rupprecht 2002). Both allopregnanolone and DHEA are also synthesized in the peripheral adrenal gland, and due to their lipophilic nature can easily cross the blood–brain barrier, thereby influencing central nervous functions and activities, including neuronal survival and differentiation, cognition, mood, sense of well-being, aggression and feeding (Rupprecht 2002). There is evidence that allopregnanolone, which is a positive modulator of gamma-aminobutyric acid (receptor A) (GABA-A) and glycine receptors, may increase feeding behavior and weight, whereas DHEA and DHEA-S, which are negative modulators of GABA-A and glycine receptors and positive modulators of glutamate and serotonin receptors, may decrease food intake and weight (Reddy and Kulkarni 1998; Pham *et al.* 2000).

Since in the adrenal glands the secretion of neuroactive steroids is driven by the CRF–ACTH system, and because of the overdrive of the HPA axis in AN, changes in circulating DHEA and DHEA-S are expected in acutely ill anorexic patients. Initial work on small patient samples provided evidence for decreased production of both DHEA and DHEA-S in underweight women with AN (Zumoff *et al.* 1983; Winterer *et al.* 1985). This reduction, together with the increase in cortisol levels, led to decreased DHEA:cortisol and DHEA-S:cortisol ratios, reflecting a dissociation in the adrenal secretion similar to that which occurs in the prepubertal stage of sexual maturation. Therefore, it was postulated that in acutely ill postpubertal anorexic patients, there is a regression to a prepubertal status of functioning which affects not only the reproductive axis, but also the HPA axis. This hypothesis was not supported by subsequent studies (Monteleone *et al.* 2001; Galderisi *et al.* 2003), which found, in underweight anorexic women, increased plasma levels of DHEA, DHEA-S and cortisol, with preservation of their ratios and positive correlations between neurosteroids and cognitive tasks also suggesting that changes in neuroactive steroids influence neurocognitive performance in eating disorders.

A recent study by Stein and colleagues (2005) measured neurosteroid levels in adolescent AN patients. No differences were shown in plasma levels of cortisol, DHEA and DHEA-S between female adolescent inpatients with restrictive AN and healthy controls. The patient group had significantly lower cortisol:DHEA-S ratios than controls, which indicates a regression of the HPA system to prepubertal functioning, as previously suggested. Moreover, cortisol levels, but not DHEA and DHEA-S levels, were decreased in the patient group after four months of weight restoration compared with admission, with a concomitant trend towards a decrease in cortisol:DHEA and cortisol:DHEA-S ratios. Since DHEA and DHEA-S tend to decrease whereas cortisol tends to increase the daily caloric intake during refeeding (Gordon *et al.* 2002), the authors speculated that the non-significant decrease in DHEA and DHEA-S levels following refeeding, in contrast to the significant reduction in cortisol levels, may account in part for the decrease in food consumption that is often observed in AN patients when they reach their desired weight.

The dynamics of neurosteroid production by the adrenal gland have been assessed by measuring changes in plasma levels of allopregnanolone and DHEA after administering 1 mg of dexamethasone at 8.00 am in underweight AN patients (Monteleone *et al.* 2006). Although AN patients had higher morning cortisol levels than healthy controls, dexamethasone efficiently suppressed cortisol secretion, and there were no significant quantitative or timing differences between the two groups. With regard to DHEA, dexamethasone significantly reduced plasma levels of the neuroactive steroid in both patients and controls, but in patients the circulating DHEA levels were significantly increased over the 24-hour study period, and reached a nadir earlier than in the latter. No major differences in allopregnanolone secretion were found between the two groups. These results led the authors to suggest that, in AN, the enhanced production of peripheral DHEA is not due merely to the increased CRF/ACTH drive since, in contrast to cortisol, circulating DHEA levels after dexamethasone administration were not reduced to the values found in control women as would have occurred after the complete inhibition of the CRF/ACTH system by administration of 1 mg of dexamethasone. Therefore, factors other than the CRF/ACTH drive, which are not affected by the exogenous corticosteroid, may contribute to the enhanced production of DHEA in AN. The nature of these factors has yet to be identified.

Brain-derived neurotrophic factor

Brain-derived neurotrophic factor (BDNF) is the most abundant neurotrophin both in the central and peripheral nervous system. It is known to exert various effects on the nervous system, promoting neuronal outgrowth and differentiation, synaptic connectivity and neuronal repair (Lewin and Barde 1996). Several lines of evidence indicate that this neurotrophin also has a role in eating behavior. Indeed, heterozygous mice with one functional BDNF allele and mice in which the BDNF gene has been deleted in excitatory brain neurons display obesity phenotypes with increased locomotor activity (Kernie *et al.* 2000). Moreover, both central and peripheral administration of BDNF decreases food intake, increases energy expenditure and ameliorates hyperinsulinemia and hyperglycemia in diabetic *db/db* mice via a central nervous system-mediated mechanism (Nagakawa *et al.* 2000; Tsuchida *et al.* 2001). In addition, BDNF and its tyrosine kinase receptor are expressed in various hypothalamic nuclei that are implicated in the regulation of eating behavior (Kernie *et al.* 2000). Collectively, these findings suggest that BDNF signaling in the brain may play a role in eating disorders.

Nakazato and colleagues (2003) reported that, compared with age-matched healthy controls, women with AN or BN (both drug-free and drug-treated) exhibited lower serum BDNF levels. This reduction was more pronounced in AN than in BN, and serum BDNF levels were negatively correlated with depressive symptoms. Monteleone and colleagues (2004b) confirmed that circulating BDNF levels were significantly reduced in drug-free underweight anorexic patients, but were increased in obese women, and they found a significant positive correlation between serum BDNF levels and body weight and body mass index.

In a study that included acutely ill drug-free patients with AN, BN or BED, serum BDNF levels were found to be significantly decreased in individuals with AN and BN, but not in those with BED (Monteleone *et al.* 2005a). Moreover, serum concentrations of BDNF did not differ significantly between AN and BN patients with or without comorbid depressive disorders, and were not correlated with severity of depressive symptomatology. This rules out the evidence that reduced levels of serum BDNF in eating-disordered patients were related to the co-occurrence of a mood disorder. Finally, decreased BDNF levels in patients with eating disorders were not secondary to malnutrition-induced changes in the estrogen and thyroid hormone milieu, since no significant correlation was found between serum BDNF and 17-estradiol, FT_3 or FT_4 levels in either AN or BN patients (Monteleone *et al.* 2005a).

Decreased circulating BDNF levels in emaciated AN patients were not restored after partial weight recovery (Nakazato *et al.* 2006). With regard to the pathophysiological significance of decreased circulating BDNF levels in eating-disordered patients, one hypothesis could be that, since BDNF exerts a satiety effect, its reduction may represent an adaptive phenomenon that aims to counteract the reduced calorie intake through increasing hunger. In addition, it has been demonstrated that mice with reduced hypothalamic BDNF expression exhibit an increase in locomotor activity (Kernie *et al.* 2000). Therefore, the possibility exists that reduced BDNF levels in women with AN or BN might sustain the increased physical activity of these patients.

Neurodevelopment

Several lines of evidence show that the prenatal period is important for understanding the etiopathogenesis of many psychiatric and non-psychiatric disorders. The intrauterine environment is crucial for the development of brain and other tissues (e.g. adipose tissue, muscle), because differentiation and replication mainly occur during limited periods (Hales and Barker 2001; Bateson 2007). Critical periods are particularly implicated in the development of neuropsychiatric disorders (because of possible interference with neurodevelopment) and metabolic and cardiovascular disorders (because of possible alterations in the programming of some important physiological and endocrinological functions). Different types of fetal exposure are considered to be possible risk factors for psychiatric disorders. These include nutritional factors (Clarke *et al.* 2006), pregnancy complications (Clarke *et al.* 2006), infectious diseases (Westergaard *et al.* 1999) and severe stress (Huizink *et al.* 2004), as well as some toxic substances (e.g. nicotine, alcohol, drugs).

Few studies to date have explored the role of intrauterine exposure in the etiopathogenesis of eating disorders (Connan *et al.* 2003; Bulik *et al.* 2005). Observation of neuropsychological deficits (Galderisi *et al.* 2003; Tchanturia *et al.* 2005), subtle neurological abnormalities and non-reversible morphological brain changes (Lask *et al.* 2005) might suggest that impairment of neurodevelopment could be one of the possible pathways to AN.

Several previous studies have revealed a high incidence of obstetric complications in AN, but only two studies, using the Swedish birth register, used a prospective design (Cnattingius *et al.* 1999; Lindberg and Hjern 2003). They found that obstetric complications might have a role in increasing the risk of developing AN, and in particular that there is a significant association with very premature birth and cephalhematoma. Obstetric complications might have more than one role in the pathogenesis of eating disorders. First, they may cause hypoxia-induced damage to the brain, which could impair the neurodevelopment of the fetus, as has been described in schizophrenia (Clarke *et al.* 2006). Secondly, the occurrence of obstetric complications might increase the mother's anxiety during and after pregnancy, and thus increase the risk of an insecure attachment (Connan *et al.* 2003). Thirdly, the adequacy of nutrition during pregnancy and in the immediate postnatal period might be implicated in the regulation of the nutritional status of the adult, and in appetite programming throughout life (Hales and Barker 2001). Nutritional factors could be particularly implicated in the case of mothers who have had an eating disorder, since recovered subjects usually maintain a lower weight (Bulik *et al.* 2006). According to Bulik and colleagues (2005), mothers with lifetime AN expose their offspring to 'a double disadvantage' – one due to the transmission of genes that increase the risk for AN, and the other due to an increased risk of inadequate nutrition and weight gain during pregnancy.

A recent prospective birth cohort study (Favaro *et al.* 2006) gave further support to these hypotheses, as it found a significant relationship between the occurrence of specific types of perinatal complication and the development of eating disorders. This study was able to differentiate between complications occurring early in pregnancy, such as anemia or pre-eclampsia, and those linked to the perinatal period, such as neonatal hyporeactivity or early respiratory or cardiac problems. This distinction is important, because early complications might influence neurodevelopment, whereas later ones might be either a cause of hypoxia and brain damage (especially in the highly vulnerable areas of the cortex and hippocampus) or effects/signs of neurodevelopmental problems. The study found that both early and late complications are significantly and independently associated with the risk of developing AN. A significant association has been found between AN and maternal anemia, diabetes, pre-eclampsia, placental infarction, neonatal cardiac problems and hyporeactivity. The study observed a dose–response effect for all obstetric complications in increasing the risk of AN, indicating a positive interaction between different types of complications. In addition, an increasing number of complications significantly anticipated the age of onset of AN. This type of relationship is considered to be evidence of a causal link, and would indicate that impairment of neurodevelopment could be implicated in the pathogenesis of AN. The study by Favaro *et al.* (2006) was the first to explore, with a prospective design, the role of obstetric complications in the development of BN. For this group, the perinatal risk factors that were significantly associated with risk of developing the disorder were placental infarction, neonatal hyporeactivity, early eating difficulties, and a low birth weight for gestational age.

Other recent studies seem to indicate a developmental origin of eating disorders. Several studies have found that patients with AN are more likely to be born during the spring months (Eagles *et al.* 2001). Various hypotheses have been proposed to explain the season-of-birth bias in AN, including seasonal variation in parental procreation habits, intrauterine infections, nutritional factors, and temperature at the time of conception. A study of the pattern of birth of individuals with early-onset AN (Willoughby *et al.* 2005) found that patients in an equatorial region do not seem to show seasonality of birth. This finding would support the importance of temperature at the time of conception. However, the 'temperature at conception' hypothesis is put in doubt by the study of Jongbloet *et al.* (2005), who found that the pattern of birth observed in AN could be better explained by the seasonal pre-ovulatory over-ripeness ovopathy and seasonal optimally ripened oocytes hypotheses. However, both studies cannot reject other explanatory hypotheses of seasonality of birth. A recent study of family composition (Eagles *et al.* 2005) found that anorexic individuals are significantly later in birth order compared with healthy subjects. The more siblings a person has while *in utero*, the more likely it is that the mother will be exposed to common infections and influenza (Westergaard *et al.* 1999), so this finding would be compatible with an infection hypothesis to explain seasonality of birth in AN.

Miscellanea

Hypothalamic–pituitary–thyroid axis

Altered hypothalamic–pituitary–thyroid function has been observed in eating disorders. Onur and colleagues (2005) found a close association between the changes in resting energy expenditure during weight gain and the increase in levels of tri-iodothyronine, even after controlling for changes in fat-free mass. The study provides further evidence that the low tri-iodothyronine levels reflect metabolic adaptation in patients with AN. Brambilla and colleagues (2006) explored the correlation of TSH, tri-iodothyronine and thyroxine levels with psychiatric and eating psychopathology in eating-disordered patients. The presence of significant correlations suggests that thyroid function may reflect or modulate the severity, consistency and persistence of psychological symptoms in eating disorders.

Agouti-related protein

Agouti-related protein is a naturally occurring antagonist of melanocortin action that is thought to play an important role in the hypothalamic control of feeding behavior. A polymorphism of the agouti-related protein gene has been associated with AN (Vink *et al.* 2001), suggesting a possible role of this protein in the pathogenesis of eating disorders. A recent study by Moriya *et al.* (2006) found increased levels of agouti-related protein in patients with AN, and a negative correlation of the protein levels with leptin and body mass index. These observations seem to suggest a role of agouti-related protein as a nutritional marker and in the abnormal energy homeostasis of patients with eating disorders (Moriya *et al.* 2006).

Endocannabinoid system

Alterations of the endocannabinoid system could be involved in the pathophysiology of eating disorders. The endocannabinoid system has been shown to control food intake in both animals and humans, modulating either rewarding or quantitative aspects of eating behavior (Cota *et al.* 2003). In addition, hypothalamic endocannabinoids seem to be part of the neural circuitry involved in the modulating effects of leptin on energy homeostasis. In a study by Monteleone *et al.* (2005d), plasma levels of the endogenous ligand anandamide were significantly enhanced in patients with AN and BED, but not in those with BN. Circulating anandamide levels were significantly and inversely correlated with plasma leptin levels in both healthy controls and women with AN. No correlation with the clinical characteristics of eating-disordered patients emerged. The findings of this study suggest the possible involvement of the endocannabinoid anandamide in the mediation of the rewarding aspects of the aberrant eating behaviors that occur in AN and BED.

Summary of important findings and future directions

This review has highlighted recent advances in various areas of neurobiological research. Neurotransmitters, such as serotonin and dopamine, showed important associations with core symptoms and behavior of eating disorders, such as anxiety, harm avoidance and impulsivity. The exploration of the functioning of hypothalamic–pituitary axes has shown interesting and useful links with body composition, pattern of weight recovery, resumption of menses, and bone loss. Studies of gastrointestinal peptides and adipokines have shown an association between the circulating levels of these peptides and alterations in food intake, satiety and motor activity in AN, BN and BED. Other interesting neurohormones and neuropeptides, such as neurosteroids and brain-derived neurotrophic factor, seem to have the function of linking or modulating different types of functions, such as neurocognition, neurodevelopment, neuroendocrinology and behavior. Further research in both acutely ill and recovered subjects is needed in order to obtain a full understanding of these complex functions and their role in the pathogenesis or maintenance of eating disorders. It is still not clear which alterations are primary and which are secondary to the presence of an eating disorder and/or to malnutrition, and this knowledge is crucial for an understanding of the pathogenesis and pathophysiology of eating disorders.

Few studies to date have explored the role of neurodevelopment as a possible pathway to eating disorders. According to a neurodevelopmental hypothesis, it would be important to understand which specific functions of the brain are impaired by obstetric complications, and how these alterations can lead to an increased risk of developing eating disorders. Future studies should address the issue of the relationship between neuroimaging and neuropsychological impairment and the presence of obstetric complications in early- and late-onset AN.

Clinical implications

Recent studies have highlighted the fact that advances in the neurobiological characteristics can be important not only for gaining new insights into the etiopathogenetic process of eating disorders, but also for understanding the pathogenesis of medical complications, such as osteoporosis. In addition, neurobiological alterations are associated with particular comorbid and behavioral traits that are considered to be of particular relevance to the planning of effective and individualized treatments. The aim of recent and future studies in this field is to provide new elements to plan more effective preventive strategies and treatment techniques. Recent findings are important, but have yet to lead to significantly improved treatments and a better outcome for patients. The aim of studies in the next decade will be to elucidate the specific neurobiological, psychological and sociocultural factors that are of etiological significance in eating disorders, and to try to translate these findings into more effective treatments.

References

(References included from the targeted review years are preceded by one asterisk. References preceded by three asterisks are of particular significance. The significance is explained by a short commentary following the complete reference.)

Adrian TE, Ferri Gl, Bacarese-Hamilton AJ, Fuessl HS, Polak JM and Bloom SR (1985) A human distribution and release of a putative new gut hormone, peptide YY. *Gastroenterology*, **89:** 1070–7.

*Asakawa A, Inui A, Fujimiya M, Sakamaki R, Shinfuku N, Ueta Y *et al.* (2005) Stomach regulates energy balance via acylated ghrelin and desacyl ghrelin. *Gut*, **54:** 18–24.

*Atchley DP and Eckel LA (2005) Fenfluramine treatment in female rats accelerates the weight loss associated with activity-based anorexia. *Pharmacology, Biochemistry and Behavior*, **80:** 273–9.

*Atchley DP and Eckel LA (2006) Treatment with 8-OH-DPAT attenuates the weight loss associated with activity-based anorexia in female rats. *Pharmacology, Biochemistry and Behavior*, **83:** 547–53.

*Bailer UF, Frank GK, Henry SE, Price JC, Meltzer CC *et al.* (2005) Altered brain serotonin 5-HT1A receptor binding after recovery from anorexia nervosa measured by positron emission tomography and [Carbonyl^{11}C]WAY-100635. *Archives of General Psychiatry*, **62:** 1032–41.

*Bailer UF, Frank GK, Henry SE, Price JC, Meltzer CC, Mathis CA *et al.* (2007) Exaggerated 5-HT1A but normal 5-HT2A receptor activity in individuals ill with anorexia nervosa. *Biological Psychiatry*, **61:** 1090–9.

Bateson P (2007) Developmental plasticity and evolutionary biology. *Journal of Nutrition*, **137:** 1060–2.

Batterham RL, Cohen MA, Ellis SM, Le Roux CW, Withers DJ, Frost GS *et al.* (2003) Inhibition of food intake in obese subject by peptide YY_{3-36}. *New England Journal of Medicine*, **349:** 941–8.

*Bergen AW, Yeager M, Welch RA, Haque K, Ganjei JK, van den Bree MBM *et al.* (2005) Association of multiple DRD2 polymorphisms with anorexia nervosa. *Neuropsychopharmacology*, **30:** 1703–19.

Berrettini WH, Kaye WH, Gwirtsmann H and Allbright A (1988) Cerebrospinal fluid peptide YY immunoreactivity in eating disorders. *Neuropsychobiology*, **19:** 121–4.

*Birketvedt GS, Drivenes E, Agledahl I, Sundsfjord J, Olstad R and Florholmen JR (2006) Bulimia nervosa – a primary defect in the hypothalamic–pituitary–adrenal axis? *Appetite*, **46:** 164–7.

Bliss E and Migeon CJ (1957) Endocrinology of anorexia nervosa. *Journal of Clinical Endocrinology and Metabolism*, **17:** 766–76.

Blundell JE, Goodson S and Halford JCG (2001) Regulation of appetite: role of leptin in signalling systems for drive and satiety. *International Journal of Obesity*, **25 (Suppl. 1):** 529–34.

*Bosy-Westphal A, Brabant G, Haas V, Onur S, Paul T, Nutzinger D *et al.* (2005) Determinants of plasma adiponectin levels in patients with anorexia nervosa examined before and after weight gain. *European Journal of Nutrition*, **44:** 355–9.

Bouloumie A, Drexler HC, Lafontan M and Busse R (1998) Leptin, the product of Ob gene, promotes angiogenesis. *Circulation Research*, **83:** 1059–66.

Brambilla F and Monteleone P (2003) Physical complications and physiological aberrations in eating disorders: a review. In: Maj M, Halmi K, Lopez-Ibor JJ and Sartorius N, editors. *Eating Disorders*. Chichester: Wiley & Sons Ltd, pp. 139–92.

Brambilla F, Bellodi L, Arancio C, Ronchi P and Limonta D (2001) Central dopaminergic function in anorexia and bulimia nervosa: a psychoneuroendocrine approach. *Psychoneuroendocrinology*, **26**: 393–409.

*Brambilla F, Santonastaso P, Caregaro L and Favaro A (2006) Disorders of eating behavior: correlation between hypothalamo–pituitary function and psychopathological aspects. *Psychoneuroendocrinology*, **31**: 131–6.

*Bruce KR, Steiger H, Ng Ying Kin NMK and Israel M (2006) Reduced platelet [³H-]paroxetine binding in anorexia nervosa: relationship to eating symptoms and personality pathology. *Psychiatry Research*, **142**: 225–32.

*Bulik CM, Reba L, Siega-Riz AM and Reichborn-Kjennerud TR (2005) Anorexia nervosa: definition, epidemiology, and cycle of risk. *International Journal of Eating Disorders*, **37**: S2–9.

Bulik CM, Sullivan PF, Tozzi F, Furberg H, Lichtenstein P and Pedersen NL (2006) Prevalence, heritability, and prospective risk factors for anorexia nervosa. *Archives of General Psychiatry*, **63**: 305–12.

*Casper RC (2006) The 'drive for activity' and 'restlessness' in anorexia nervosa: potential pathways. *Journal of Affective Disorders*, **92**: 99–107.

*Castro-Fornieles J, Deulofeu R, Baeza I, Casulà V, Saura B, Lazaro L et al. (2006) Psychopathological and nutritional correlates of plasma homovanillic acid in adolescents with anorexia nervosa. *Journal of Psychiatric Research*, (e-publication ahead of print).

***Chan JL and Mantzoros CS (2005) Role of leptin in energy-deprivation states: normal human physiology and clinical implications for hypothalamic amenorrhoea and anorexia nervosa. *Lancet*, **366**: 74–85.

This is an excellent and well-written review about the normal physiology of leptin and its role in signalling energy availability in energy-deficient states. The review showed that low concentrations of leptin are fully or partly responsible for starvation-induced changes in neuroendocrine axes, including low reproductive, thyroid and insulin-like growth factor (IGF) hormones.

*Chen CY, Inui A, Asakawa A, Fujino K, Kato I, Chen CC et al. (2005) Des-acyl ghrelin acts by CRF type 2 receptors to disrupt fasted stomach motility in conscious rats. *Gastroenterology*, **129**: 8–25.

Clarke MC, Harley M and Cannon M (2006) The role of obstetric events in schizophrenia. *Schizophrenia Bulletin*, **32**: 3–8.

Cnattingius S, Hultman CM, Dahl M and Sparen P (1999) Very preterm birth, birth trauma, and the risk of anorexia nervosa among girls. *Archives of General Psychiatry*, **56**: 634–8.

Connan F, Campbell IC, Katzman M, Lightman SL and Treasure J (2003) A neurodevelopmental model for anorexia nervosa. *Physiology and Behavior*, **79**: 13–24.

Cota D, Marsicano G, Lutz B, Vicennati V, Stalla GK, Pasquali R et al. (2003) Endogenous cannabinoid system as a modulator of food intake. *International Journal of Obesity and Related Metabolic Disorders*, **27**: 289–301.

Cummings DE, Purnell JQ, Frayo RS, Schmidova K, Wisse BE and Weigle DS (2001) A preprandial rise in plasma ghrelin levels suggests a role in meal initiation in humans. *Diabetes*, **50**: 1714–19.

Delporte ML, Brichard SM, Hermans MP, Beguin C and Lambert M (2003) Hyperadiponectinaemia in anorexia nervosa. *Clinical Endocrinology*, **58**: 22–9.

Di Chiara G (1999) Drug addiction as dopamine-dependent associative learning disorder. *European Journal of Pharmacology*, **375**: 13–30.

*Dostalova I, Kopsky V, Duskova J, Papezova H, Pacak K and Nedvidkova J (2005) Leptin concentrations in the abdominal subcutaneous adipose tissue of patients with anorexia nervosa assessed by *in vivo* microdialysis. *Regulatory Peptides*, **128**: 63–8.

*Dostalova I, Smitka K, Papezova H, Kvasnickova H and Nedvidkova J (2006a) Increased insulin sensitivity in patients with anorexia nervosa: the role of adipocytokines. *Physiological Research*, Dec 19 (Epub ahead of print).

*Dostalova I, Kunesova M, Duskova J, Papezova H and Nedvidkova J (2006b) Adipose tissue resistin levels in patients with anorexia nervosa. *Nutrition*, **22**: 977–83.

Druce MR, Small CJ and Bloom SR (2004) Minireview: Gut peptides regulating satiety. *Endocrinology*, **145**: 2660–5.

Eagles JM, Andrew JE, Johnston MI, Easton EA and Millar HR (2001) Season of birth in females with anorexia nervosa in northeast Scotland. *International Journal of Eating Disorders*, **30**: 167–75.

*Eagles JM, Johnston MI and Millar HR (2005) A case–control study of family composition in anorexia nervosa. *International Journal of Eating Disorders*, **38**: 49–54.

Exner C, Hebebrand J, Remschmidt H, Wewetzer C, Ziegler A, Herpertz S *et al.* (2000) Leptin suppresses semi-starvation-induced hyperactivity in rats: implications for anorexia nervosa. *Molecular Psychiatry*, **5**: 476–81.

Fantuzzi G and Faggioni R (2000) Leptin in the regulation of immunity, inflammation and haematopoiesis. *Journal of Leukocyte Biology*, **68**: 437–46.

***Favaro A, Tenconi E and Santonastaso P (2006) Perinatal factors and the risk of developing anorexia nervosa and bulimia nervosa. *Archives of General Psychiatry*, **63**: 82–8.

This birth cohort study found that several obstetric complications, such as pre-eclampsia, diabetes, neonatal hyporeactivity and cardiac problems, significantly increase the risk of developing anorexia nervosa. The number of perinatal complications was inversely correlated with age of onset. Placental infarction, neonatal hyporeactivity, early eating difficulties and a low birth weight for gestational age were significant predictors of bulimia nervosa.

*Frank GK, Boiler UF, Henry SE, Drevets W, Meltzer CC, Price JC *et al.* (2005) Increased dopamine D2/D3 receptor binding after recovery from anorexia nervosa measured by positron emission tomography and [^{11}C]raclopride. *Biological Psychiatry*, **58**: 908–12.

Galderisi S, Mucci A, Monteleone P, Sorrentino D, Piegari G and Maj M (2003) Neurocognitive functioning in subjects with eating disorders: the influence of neuroactive steroids. *Biological Psychiatry*, **53**: 921–7.

*Golden NH, Iglesias E, Jacobson MS, Carey D, Meyer W, Schebendach J *et al.* (2005) Aledronate for the treatment of osteopenia in anorexia nervosa: a randomized, double-blind, placebo-controlled trial. *Journal of Clinical Endocrinology and Metabolism*, **90**: 3179–85.

Gordon CM, Grace E, Emans SJ, Feldman H, Goodman E, Becker KA *et al.* (2002) Effects of oral dehydroepiandrosterone on bone density in young women with anorexia nervosa: a randomized trial. *Journal of Clinical Endocrinology and Metabolism*, **87**: 4935–41.

Grinspoon S, Miller K, Coyle C, Krempin J, Armstrong C, Pitts S *et al.* (1999) Severity of osteopenia in oestrogen-deficient women with anorexia nervosa and hypothalamic amenorrhea. *Journal of Clinical Endocrinology and Metabolism*, **84**: 2049–55.

*Haas V, Onur S, Paul T, Nutzinger DO, Bosy-Westphal A and Hauer M (2005) Leptin and body weight regulation in patients with anorexia nervosa before and during weight recovery. *American Journal of Clinical Nutrition*, **81**: 889–96.

Hales CN and Barker DJ (2001) The thrifty phenotype hypothesis. *British Medical Bulletin*, **60**: 5–20.

Havel PJ (2002) Control of energy homeostasis and insulin action by adipocyte hormones: leptin, acylation-stimulating protein and adiponectin. *Current Opinion in Lipidology*, **13**: 51–9.

Hebebrand J, Exner C, Hebebrand K, Holtkamp C, Casper RC, Remschmidt H *et al.* (2003) Hyperactivity in patients with anorexia nervosa and in semi-starved rats: evidence for a pivotal role of hypoleptinemia. *Physiology and Behavior*, **79**: 25–37.

*Hillebrand JJ, Koeners MP, de Rijke CE, Kas MJ and Adan RA (2005) Leptin treatment in activity-based anorexia. *Biological Psychiatry*, **58**: 165–71.

Holtkamp K, Hebebrand J, Mika C, Grzella I, Heer M, Heussen N *et al.* (2003) The effect of therapeutically induced weight gain on plasma leptin levels in patients with anorexia nervosa. *Journal of Psychiatric Research*, **37**: 165–9.

Holtkamp K, Hebebrand J, Mika C, Heer M, Heussen N and Herpertz-Dahlmann B (2004) High serum leptin levels subsequent to weight gain predict renewed weight loss in patients with anorexia nervosa. *Psychoneuroendocrinology*, **29**: 791–7.

*Holtkamp K, Herpertz-Dahlmann B, Hebebrand K, Mika C, Kratzsch J and Hebebrand J (2006) Physical activity and restlessness correlate with leptin levels in patients with adolescent anorexia nervosa. *Biological Psychiatry*, **60**: 311–13.

*Housova J, Anderlova K, Krizova J, Haluzikova D, Kremen J, Kumstyrova T *et al.* (2005) Serum adiponectin and resistin concentrations in patients with restrictive and binge/purge form of anorexia nervosa and bulimia nervosa. *Journal of Clinical Endocrinology and Metabolism*, **90**: 1366–70.

Huizink AC, Mulder EJH and Buitelaar JK (2004) Prenatal stress and risk for psychopathology: specific effects or induction of general susceptibility? *Psychological Bulletin*, **130**: 115–42.

Iwahashi H, Funahashi T, Kurokawa N, Sayama K, Fukuda E, Okita K *et al.* (2003) Plasma adiponectin levels in women with anorexia nervosa. *Hormone and Metabolic Research*, **35**: 537–40.

*Janas-Kozik M, Krupka-Matuszczyk I, Malinowska-Kolodziej I and Lewin-Kowalik J (2007) Total ghrelin plasma level in patients with the restrictive type of anorexia nervosa. *Regulatory Peptides*, **140**: 43–6

Jimerson DC and Wolfe BE (2004) Neuropeptides in eating disorders. *CNS Spectrum*, **9**: 516–22.

Jimerson DC and Wolfe BE (2006) Psychobiology of eating disorders. In: Wonderlich S, Mitchell JE, de Zwaan M and Steiger H, editors. *Annual Review of Eating Disorders*. Oxford: Radcliffe Publishing, pp. 1–16.

*Jongbloet PH, Groenewoud HMM and Roeleveld N (2005) Seasonally bound ovopathy versus 'temperature at conception' as cause for anorexia nervosa and other eating disorders. *International Journal of Eating Disorders*, **38**: 236–43.

Kaye WH, Berrettini W, Gwirtsman H and George DT (1990) Altered cerebrospinal fluid neuropeptide Y and peptide YY immunoreactivity in anorexia and bulimia nervosa. *Archives of General Psychiatry*, **47**: 548–56.

*Kaye WH, Frank GK, Bailer UF and Henry SE (2005a) Neurobiology of anorexia nervosa: clinical implications of alterations of the function of serotonin and other neuronal systems. *International Journal of Eating Disorders*, **37**: S15–19.

*Kaye WH, Frank GK, Bailer UF, Henry SE, Meltzer CC, Price JC *et al.* (2005b) Serotonin alterations in anorexia and bulimia nervosa: new insights from imaging studies. *Physiology and Behavior*, **85**: 73–81.

Kernie SG, Liebl DJ and Parada LF (2000) BDNF regulates eating behavior and locomotor activity in mice. *EMBO Journal*, **19**: 1290–300.

*Kojima S, Nakahara T, Nagai N, Muranaga T, Tanaka M, Yasuhara D *et al.* (2005) Altered ghrelin and peptide YY responses to meals in bulimia nervosa. *Clinical Endocrinology*, **62**: 74–8.

Lask B, Gordon I, Christie D, Frampton I, Chowdhury U and Watkins B (2005) Functional neuroimaging in early-onset anorexia nervosa. *International Journal of Eating Disorders,* **37:** S49–51.

Lewin GR and Barde YA (1996) Physiology of neurotrophins. *Annual Review of Neuroscience,* **19:** 289–317.

Lieberman UA, Weis SR, Broll J, Minne HW, Quan H, Bell NH *et al.* (1995) Effect of oral aledronate on bone mineral density and the incidence of fractures in postmenopausal osteoporosis. The Aledronate Phase III Osteoporosis Treatment Study Group. *New England Journal of Medicine,* **333:** 1437–43.

Lindberg L and Hjern A (2003) Risk factors for anorexia nervosa: a national cohort study. *International Journal of Eating Disorders,* **34:** 397–408.

*Miller KK, Grieco KA and Klibanski A (2005) Testosterone administration in women with anorexia nervosa. *Journal of Clinical Endocrinology and Metabolism,* **90:** 1428–33.

***Misra M, Miller KK, Almazan C, Worley M, Herzog DB and Klibanski A (2005a) Hormonal determinants of regional body composition in adolescent girls with anorexia nervosa and controls. *Journal of Clinical Endocrinology and Metabolism,* **90:** 2580–7.
This study explored the effects of endocrine alterations on regional body composition in 23 adolescent girls with AN and 20 healthy girls. It was found that in healthy controls, GH concentration predicts regional body composition and favors a redistribution of body fat. However, in AN the presence of high levels of both GH and cortisol has contrasting effects. High cortisol levels in AN predict a redistribution of lean body mass such that extremity lean mass decreases.

*Misra M, Miller KK, Kuo K, Griffin K, Stewart V, Hunter E *et al.* (2005b) Secretory dynamics of leptin in adolescent girls with anorexia nervosa and healthy adolescents. *American Journal of Physiology – Endocrinology and Metabolism,* **289:** 373–81.

*Misra M, Prabhakaran R, Miller KK, Tsai P, Lin A, Lee N *et al.* (2006a) Role of cortisol in menstrual recovery in adolescent girls with anorexia nervosa. *Pediatric Research,* **59:** 598–603.

*Misra M, Miller KK, Tsai P, Gallagher K, Lin A, Lee N *et al.* (2006b) Elevated peptide YY levels in adolescent girls with anorexia nervosa. *Journal of Clinical Endocrinology and Metabolism,* **91:** 1027–33.

*Mondelli V, Gianotti L, Picu A, Abbate Daga G, Giordano R, Berardelli R *et al.* (2006) Neuroendocrine effects of citalopram infusion in anorexia nervosa. *Psychoneuroendocrinology,* **31:** 1139–48.

Monteleone P, Luisi M, Colurcio B, Casarosa E, Monteleone P, Ioime R *et al.* (2001) Plasma levels of neuroactive steroids are increased in untreated women with anorexia nervosa or bulimia nervosa. *Psychosomatic Medicine,* **63:** 62–8.

Monteleone P, Fabrazzo M, Martiadis V, Fuschino A, Serritella C, Milici N *et al.* (2003) Opposite changes in circulating adiponectin in women with bulimia nervosa or binge eating disorder. *Journal of Clinical Endocrinology and Metabolism,* **88:** 5387–91.

Monteleone P, Di Lieto A, Castaldo E and Maj M (2004a) Leptin functioning in eating disorders. *CNS Spectrum,* **9:** 523–9.

Monteleone P, Tortorella A, Martiadis V, Serritella C, Fuschino A and Maj M (2004b) Opposite changes in the serum brain-derived neurotrophic factor in anorexia nervosa and obesity. *Psychosomatic Medicine,* **66:** 744–8.

*Monteleone P, Fabrazzo M, Martiadis V, Serritella C, Pannuto M and Maj M (2005a) Circulating brain-derived neurotrophic factor is decreased in women with anorexia and bulimia nervosa but not in women with binge-eating disorder: relationships to co-morbid depression, psychopathology and hormonal variables. *Psychological Medicine,* **35:** 897–905.

*Monteleone P, Fabrazzo M, Tortorella A, Martiadis V, Serritella C and Maj M (2005b) Circulating ghrelin is decreased in non-obese and obese women with binge-eating disorder as well as in obese non-binge-eating women, but not in patients with bulimia nervosa. *Psychoneuroendocrinology*, **30:** 243–50.

*Monteleone P, Martiadis V, Rigamonti AE, Fabrazzo M, Giordani C, Muller EE *et al.* (2005c) Investigation of peptide YY and ghrelin responses to a test meal in bulimia nervosa. *Biological Psychiatry*, **57:** 926–31.

***Monteleone P, Matias I, Martiadis V, De Petrocellis L, Maj M and Di Marzo V (2005d) Blood levels of the endocannabinoid anandamide are increased in anorexia nervosa and in binge-eating disorder, but not in bulimia nervosa. *Neuropsychopharmacology*, **30:** 1216–21.

This is the first study to explore the issue of endocannabinoids in eating disorders. The authors found that plasma levels of the endogenous ligand anandamide were significantly enhanced in patients with AN and BED, but not in those with BN. The findings suggest the possible involvement of the endocannabinoid anandamide in mediating the rewarding aspects of the aberrant eating behaviors that occur in AN and BED.

*Monteleone P, Luisi M, Martiadis V, Serritella C, Longobardi N, Casarosa E *et al.* (2006) Impaired reduction of enhanced levels of dehydroepiandrosterone by oral dexamethasone in anorexia nervosa. *Psychoneuroendocrinology*, **31:** 537–42.

*Moriya J, Takimoto Y, Yoshiuchi K, Shimosawa T and Akabayashi A (2006) Plasma agouti-related protein levels in women with anorexia nervosa. *Psychoneuroendocrinology*, **31:** 1057–61.

Moschos S, Chan JL and Mantzoros CS (2002) Leptin and reproduction: a review. *Fertility and Sterility*, **77:** 433–44.

*Naessén S, Carlstrom K, Glant R, Jacobsson H and Hirschberg AL (2006) Bone mineral density in bulimic women – influence of endocrine factors and previous anorexia. *European Journal of Endocrinology*, **155:** 245–51.

Nagakawa T, Tsuchida A, Itakura Y, Nonomura T, Ono M, Hirota F *et al.* (2000) Brain-derived neurotrophic factor regulates glucose metabolism by modulating energy balance in diabetic mice. *Diabetes*, **49:** 436–44.

*Nakahara T, Kojima S, Tanaka M, Yasuhara D, Harada T, Sagiyama KI *et al.* (2007) Incomplete restoration of the secretion of ghrelin and PYY compared to insulin after food ingestion following weight gain in anorexia nervosa. *Journal of Psychiatric Research*, **41:** 814–20.

Nakazato M, Hashimoto K, Shimizu E, Kumakiri C, Koizumi H, Okamura N *et al.* (2003) Decreased levels of serum brain-derived neurotrophic factor in female patients with eating disorders. *Biological Psychiatry*, **54:** 485–90.

*Nakazato M, Hashimoto K, Yoshimura K, Hashimoto T, Shimizu E and Iyo M (2006) No change between the serum brain-derived neurotrophic factor in female patients with anorexia nervosa before and after partial weight recovery. *Progress in Neuro-Psychopharmacology and Biological Psychiatry*, **30:** 1117–21.

Newton Jr, Preeman CP, Hannan WJ and Cowe S (1993) Osteoporosis and normal weight bulimia – which patients are at risk? *Journal of Psychosomatic Research*, **37:** 239–47.

*Onur S, Haas V, Bosy-Westphal A, Hauer M, Paul T, Nutzinger D *et al.* (2005) L-tri-iodothyronine is a major determinant of resting energy expenditure in underweight patients with anorexia nervosa and during weight gain. *European Journal of Endocrinology*, **152:** 179–84.

Otto B, Tschop M and Cuntz U (2004) Similar fasting ghrelin levels in binge-eating/purging anorexia nervosa and restrictive anorexia nervosa. *Psychoneuroendocrinology*, **29:** 692–3.

*Otto B, Tschop M, Fruhauf E, Heldwein W, Fichter M, Otto C *et al.* (2005) Postprandial ghrelin release in anorectic patients before and after weight gain. *Psychoneuroendocrinology*, **30**: 577–81.

Pannacciulli N, Vettor R, Milan G, Granzotto M, Catucci A and Federspil G (2003) Anorexia nervosa is characterized by increased adiponectin plasma levels and reduced non-oxidative glucose metabolism. *Journal of Clinical Endocrinology and Metabolism*, **88**: 1748–52.

Patel L, Buckels AC, Kinghorn IJ, Murdock PR, Holbrook JD, Plumpton C *et al.* (2003) Resistin is expressed in human macrophages and directly regulated by PPAR activators. *Biochemical and Biophysical Research Communications*, **300**: 472–6.

Pham J, Porter J, Svec D, Eiswirth C and Svec F (2000) The effect of dehydroepiandrosterone on Zucker rats selected for fat food preference. *Physiology and Behavior*, **70**: 431–41.

Qi Y, Takahashi N, Hileman SM, Patel HR, Berg AH, Pajvani UB *et al.* (2004) Adiponectin acts in the brain to decrease body weight. *Nature Medicine*, **10**: 524–9.

Reddy DS and Kulkarni SK (1998) The role of GABA-A and mitochondrial diazepam-binding inhibitor receptor on the effects of neurosteroids on food intake in mice. *Psychopharmacology*, **137**: 391–400.

Rupprecht R (2002) Neuroactive steroids: mechanism of action and neuropsychopharmacological properties. *Psychoneuroendocrinology* **28**: 139–68.

Saketos M, Sharma N and Santoro N (1993) Suppression of the hypothalamic–pituitary–ovarian axis in normal women by glucocorticoids. *Biology of Reproduction*, **49**: 1270–6.

*Schule C, Sighart C, Hennig J and Laakman G (2006) Mirtazapine inhibits cortisol concentrations in anorexia nervosa. *Progress in Neuro-Psychopharmacology and Biological Psychiatry*, **30**: 1015–19.

Soyka LA, Misra M, Frenchman A, Miller K, Grinspoon S, Schoenfeld DA *et al.* (2002) Abnormal bone mineral accrual in adolescent girls with anorexia nervosa. *Journal of Clinical Endocrinology and Metabolism*, **87**: 4177–85.

Steiger H, Koerner NM, Engleberg M, Israel M, Ng Ying Kin NMK and Young SN (2001) Self-destructiveness and serotonin function in bulimia nervosa. *Psychiatry Research*, **103**: 15–26.

Steiger H, Gauvin L, Israel M, Ng Ying Kin NMK, Young SN and Roussin J (2004) Serotonin function, personality trait variations and childhood abuse in women with bulimia-spectrum eating disorders. *Journal of Clinical Psychiatry*, **65**: 830–7.

***Steiger H, Gauvin L, Joober R, Israel M, Ng Ying Kin NMK, Bruce KR *et al.* (2006) Intrafamilial correspondences on platelet [^{3}H-]paroxetine-binding indices in bulimic probands and their unaffected first-degree relatives. *Neuropsychopharmacology*, **31**: 1785–92.

This study investigated platelet [3H-]paroxetine binding in women with bulimia nervosa, controls, and their mothers and sisters. Bulimic probands, their mothers and their sisters all displayed a significantly lower density (Bmax) of platelet–paroxetine binding than did 'control' probands, mothers and sisters. These findings suggest a heritable trait, linked to 5-HT activity, and carried by BN sufferers and their first-degree relatives.

*Stein D, Maayan R, Ram A, Loewenthal R, Achiron A, Modan-Moses D *et al.* (2005) Circulatory neurosteroid levels in underweight female adolescent anorexia nervosa inpatients following weight restoration. *European Neuropsychopharmacology*, **15**: 647–53.

Steppan CM, Bailey ST, Bhat S, Brown EJ, Banerjee RR, Wright CM *et al.* (2001) The hormone resistin links obesity to diabetes. *Nature*, **409**: 307–12.

*Stock S, Leichner P, Wong AC, Ghatei MA, Kieffer TJ, Bloom SR *et al.* (2005) Ghrelin, peptide YY, glucose-dependent insulinotropic polypeptide, and hunger responses to a mixed meal in anorexic, obese and control female adolescents. *Journal of Clinical Endocrinology and Metabolism*, **90**: 2161–8.

Tagami T, Satoh N, Usui T, Yamada K, Shimatsu A and Kuzuya H (2004) Adiponectin in anorexia nervosa and bulimia nervosa. *Journal of Clinical Endocrinology and Metabolism*, **89**: 1833–7.

Tanaka M, Naruo T, Muranaga T, Yasuhara D, Shiiya T, Nakazato M *et al.* (2002) Increased fasting plasma ghrelin levels in patients with bulimia nervosa. *European Journal of Endocrinology*, **146**: 1–3.

Tanaka M, Narau T, Nagai N, Kuroki N, Shiiya T, Nakazato M *et al.* (2003a) Habitual binge/purge behavior influences circulating ghrelin levels in eating disorders. *Journal of Psychiatric Research*, **37**: 17–22.

Tanaka M, Naruo T, Yasuhara D, Tatebe Y, Nagai N, Shiiya T *et al.* (2003b) Fasting plasma ghrelin levels in subtypes of anorexia nervosa. *Psychoneuroendocrinology*, **28**: 829–35.

Tchanturia K, Campell IC, Morris R and Treasure J (2005) Neuropsychological studies in anorexia nervosa. *International Journal of Eating Disorders*, **37**: S72–6.

*Troisi A, Di Lorenzo G, Lega I, Tesauro M, Bertoli A, Leo R *et al.* (2005) Plasma ghrelin in anorexia, bulimia and binge-eating disorder: relations with eating patterns and circulating concentrations of cortisol and thyroid hormones. *Neuroendocrinology*, **81**: 259–66.

Tsuchida A, Nonomura T, Ono-Kishino M, Nakagawa T, Taiji M and Noguchi H (2001) Acute effects of brain-derived neurotrophic factor on energy expenditure in obese diabetic mice. *International Journal of Obesity and Related Metabolic Disorders*, **25**: 1286–93.

*Uehara T, Omori I, Nakamura K, Suda M, Hosoda Y, Minegishi T *et al.* (2005) Plasma des-acyl and acyl ghrelin in patients with eating disorders. *Eating and Weight Disorders*, **10**: 264–6.

Vink T, Hinney A, van Elburg AA, van Goozen SH, Sandkuijl LA, Sinke RJ *et al.* (2001) Association between an agouti-related protein gene polymorphism and anorexia nervosa. *Molecular Psychiatry*, **6**: 325–8.

Westergaard T, Mortensen PB, Pedersen CB, Wohlfahrt J and Melbye M (1999) Exposure to prenatal and childhood infections and the risk of schizophrenia. *Archives of General Psychiatry*, **56**: 993–8.

*Willoughby K, Bowen R, Lee EL, Pathy P and Lask B (2005) Pattern of birth in early-onset anorexia nervosa: an equatorial study. *International Journal of Eating Disorders*, **37**: 61–4.

Winterer J, Gwirtsman HE, George DT, Kaye WH, Loriaux DL and Cutler GB (1985) Adrenocorticotropin-stimulated adrenal androgen secretion in anorexia nervosa: impaired secretion at low weight with normalization after long-term weight recovery. *Journal of Clinical Endocrinology and Metabolism*, **61**: 693–7.

Zipfel S, Seibel MJ, Löwe B, Beumont PJ, Kasperk C and Herzog W (2001) Osteoporosis in eating disorders: a follow-up study of patients with anorexia nervosa and bulimia nervosa. *Journal of Clinical Endocrinology and Metabolism*, **86**: 5227–33.

Zumoff B, Walsh BT, Katz JL, Levin J, Rosenfeld RJ, Kream J *et al.* (1983). Subnormal plasma dehydroisoandrosterone to cortisol ratio in anorexia nervosa: a second hormonal parameter of ontogenic regression. *Journal of Clinical Endocrinology and Metabolism*, **56**: 668–72.

2

Genetics of eating disorders

Kristen M Culbert, Jennifer D Slane and Kelly L Klump

Abstract

Objectives of review. This review summarizes twin and genetic studies of eating disorders (EDs) published in 2005 and 2006.

Summary of recent findings. Twin studies highlight important gender differences in genetic liability to ED symptoms and possible shared genetic transmission between EDs and anxiety disorders. Association and linkage analyses have suggested the presence of distinct genetic risk factors for anorexia nervosa (AN) and bulimia nervosa (BN). Serotonin and brain-derived neurotrophic factor (BDNF) genes appear to be the most promising genes for understanding susceptibility to AN and phenotypic variability within BN.

Future directions. Future studies would benefit from the continued use of narrowly defined phenotypes, quantitative traits and larger sample sizes. Additional research examining multiple polymorphisms per gene, gene x gene interactions, gene x environment interactions, and the functional significance of susceptibility genes is critically needed.

Introduction

Until recently, theories on the etiology of the eating disorders (EDs) emphasized psychosocial (e.g. sociocultural) factors. Although such factors are clearly of etiological relevance, several findings have highlighted the importance of genetic factors as well. Genetic findings from 2003 and 2004 were eloquently reviewed by Mazzeo *et al.* (2006) in the last edition of the *Annual Review of Eating Disorders*. These authors concluded that there are likely to be gender- and development-specific genetic risk factors for EDs that may contribute to the disorders' characteristic epidemiological patterns (i.e. much more prevalent in females and after puberty). Moreover, although there were insufficient data to allow unequivocal labeling of any gene as a 'risk' gene, Mazzeo *et al.* (2006) noted that the studies provided preliminary evidence for the importance of serotonin and brain-derived neurotrophic factor (BDNF) genes, and for incorporating quantitative traits (e.g. eating disorder symptoms, levels of impulsivity, anxiety, etc.) into analyses.

The purpose of the current review is to focus on the most promising twin and genetic findings from 2005 and 2006 and to identify directions for future research. Although our review focuses on anorexia nervosa (AN), bulimia nervosa (BN) and binge-eating disorder (BED), the vast majority of studies have only examined AN and BN. These data support several of the conclusions drawn by Mazzeo et al. (2006), and provide new insights into the biological systems and genes that confer risk for EDs.

Twin studies

Twin studies remain invaluable for elucidating genetic contributions to EDs, as they identify relevant traits and systems to be examined in molecular genetic studies. Past studies indicate that EDs and ED symptoms are at least moderately heritable (for a review, see Bulik et al. 2000). Current research continues to attest to genetic influences on disordered eating, as two studies found evidence for moderate heritability of cognitive dietary restraint (de Castro and Lilenfeld 2005; Tholin et al. 2005). Findings for other ED characteristics (e.g. emotional eating, hunger) were more mixed (de Castro and Lilenfeld 2005; Tholin et al. 2005), although larger ED twin studies have shown significant genetic effects on these traits as well (Bulik et al. 1998; de Castro 1999).

Twin researchers have also begun to examine the nature of genetic risk and its manifestations. Gender differences are becoming a popular area of investigation (see Mazzeo et al. 2006). Gender differences in the heritability of intentional weight loss (IWL), defined as weight loss of ≥ 5 kg, were observed in young adult female (heritability = 68%) and male (heritability = 38%) twins (Keski-Rahkonen et al. 2005). These differential genetic effects were not related to differences in BMI, and thus may have important implications for studies investigating genes for EDs. Susceptibility genes may be involved in biological systems that show gender differences. However, gender similarities in genetic effects on other ED traits have been observed (for a review, see Mazzeo et al. 2006), suggesting the need for additional studies to identify the traits that are most likely to be gender differentiated.

In addition to gender effects, twin studies have examined shared genetic transmission between EDs and related phenotypes in order to identify the nature of genetic risk. Keel et al. (2005) found evidence for shared genetic transmission between EDs and anxiety disorders in adolescent monozygotic (MZ) female twins. These findings are remarkably consistent with previous results (e.g. Bulik et al. 2001) and indicate that the genetic diathesis for EDs may be associated with the genes involved in anxiety.

Molecular genetic studies

Molecular genetic studies use linkage or association (i.e. case–control or within-family) designs to identify chromosomal regions and genes that contribute to disorders (for a review of these methods, see Klump and Gobrogge, 2005 or Mazzeo *et al.* 2006). These studies have traditionally examined genes for disorders defined categorically, an approach that results in lower statistical power and more heterogeneous phenotypes for analyses. Quantitative traits are now being incorporated into analyses in an effort to narrow phenotypes and enhance statistical power for detecting significant effects.

Linkage studies

Only one linkage study of EDs has been conducted in the last two years. Bacanu *et al.* (2005) examined evidence for linkage in families with AN and BN by incorporating six quantitative traits (obsessionality, age at menarche, anxiety, lifetime minimum BMI, concern over mistakes, and food-related obsessions) (for trait selection methods, see Bulik *et al.* 2005) into analyses. Their findings confirmed those obtained previously by suggesting that regions on chromosomes 1, 4, 10, 11, 13 and 14 may be important for EDs. Interestingly, distinct linkage signals were observed for AN and BN, with some overlap between chromosomal regions for BN and regions previously linked to obesity (e.g. chromosome 10; Bulik *et al.* 2003).

Association studies

Approximately twice the number of candidate gene studies published in 2003 and 2004 (Mazzeo *et al.* 2006) were published in 2005 and 2006 (*see* Table 1). The majority of studies examined AN or BN, and only two studies (Monteleone *et al.* 2006b, 2006c) investigated BED. However, even for AN and BN, only a small number of studies per gene exist, and findings continue to be quite mixed (see, for example, the results for cholecystokinin and catechol-O-methyltransferase in Table 1). More consistent results have been obtained for serotonin and BDNF genes.

Serotonin genes

Genes involved in the serotonin system have been most extensively studied. Serotonin is a key neurotransmitter implicated in the control of appetite and mood, and evidence has suggested serotonergic disturbances in EDs (Jimerson and Wolfe 2006). Although data for most serotonin genes are either inconsistent or insufficient to allow conclusions to be drawn (see serotonin 2c receptor, serotonin 1D receptor and serotonin 1Dβ receptor in Table 1), past and current

Table 1 Summary of association studies

| Gene | Case–control/association studies | | | | Quantitative traits | | | | | |
| | Anorexia nervosa | | Bulimia nervosa | | Anorexia nervosa | | | Bulimia nervosa | | |
	No. sig./no. conducted	Range of n	No. sig./no. conducted	Range of n	No. sig./no. conducted	Range of n	Trait	No. sig./no. conducted	Range of n	Trait
Systems involved in food intake and mood										
Serotonin 2a receptor	1/1	132	0/1	33	1/1	132	↑Harm avoidance (HA) ↓Reward dependence (RD)	1/1	33	↑Non-planning ↑Impulsivity (IMPULS)
Serotonin 2c receptor	0/0	–	0/0	–	1/1	46	↑Global Severity Index (GSI)[a] ↑Distress (DIST)[a]	1/1	36	↑GSI[a] ↑DIST[a] ↑Somatization ↑Obsessive-compulsiveness ↑Depression ↑Anxiety ↑Hostility ↑Phobic anxiety ↑Paranoid ideation

Serotonin transporter	0/1	132	1/1	24–178	2/2	21–46	↑ DIST[a] ↑ Drive for thinness (DT)[a] ↑ Body dissatisfaction* (BD)	4/5	24–178	↑ DIST[a] ↑ DT[a] ↑ BD* ↑ Anxiety ↓ BMI ↑ HA ↑ Affective instability ↑ Insecure attachment ↑ IMPULS Comorbid BPD
Serotonin 1D receptor	1[b]/1	226	0/0	–	0/0	–	–	0/0	–	–
Serotonin 1Dβ receptor	0/0	–	0/0	–	0/0	–	–	1/1	165	OCD severity Minimum BMI
Brain-derived neurotrophic factor	2/5	81–359	3/5	80–126	3/3	81–271	↑ Onset age ↑ EAT score ↓ Minimum BMI	1/2	94–126	↑ BITE score ↑ HA ↓ Minimum BMI
Systems involved in food intake and/or energy balance										
Agouti-related protein	1/1	114	0/0	–	1/1	114	↓ Interpersonal distrust	0/0	–	–
B3 adrenergic receptor	0*/1	96	0*/1	116	0/0	–	–	0/0	–	–
Cholecystokinin	1/2	96–165	0/1	116	0/0	–	–	0/0	–	–
Ghrelin receptor	0*/1	96	1/1	116	0/0	–	–	0/0	–	–

Table 1 Continued

| Gene | Case–control/association studies | | | | Quantitative traits | | | | | |
| | Anorexia nervosa | | Bulimia nervosa | | Anorexia nervosa | | | Bulimia nervosa | | |
	No. sig./no. conducted	Range of n	No. sig./no. conducted	Range of n	No. sig./no. conducted	Range of n	Trait	No. sig./no. conducted	Range of n	Trait
Ghrelin/obestatin preprohormone	1/4	114–228	2/3	108–114	1/1	114	↓ Minimum BMI ↑ Onset age	0/0	–	–
Melanocortin 3 receptor	0*/1	158	0/0	–	0/0	–	–	0/0	–	–
Systems involved in insulin response										
Adiponectin	0/1	17	0/0	–	0/0	–	–	0/0	–	–
Resistin	1/1	17	0/0	–	0/0	–	–	0/0	–	–
Systems involved in pleasure and reward										
Catechol-O-methyltransferase	1/2	52–91	1*/1	28	1/1	21	↑ Bulimia score[a] ↑ Ineffectiveness[a] ↑ Interoceptive awareness[a] ↑ Maturity fears[a] ↑ Impulse regulation[a]	1[a]/1	24	↑ Bulimia score[a] ↑ Ineffectiveness[a] ↑ Interoceptive awareness[a] ↑ Maturity fears[a] ↑ Impulse regulation[a]
Dopamine transporter	0/1	91	0/0	–	0/0	–	–	0/0	–	–

Dopamine D2 receptor	1/1	191	0/0	–	0/0	–	0/0	–
Opioid delta receptor	1c/1	226	0/0	–	0/0	–	0/0	–
Miscellaneous systems								
Calcium-activated potassium channel	1/1	90	0/0	–	0/0	–	0/0	–
N-methyl-D-aspartate receptor 2B	1c/1	90	0/0	–	0/0	–	0/0	–

Note: Genes are arranged according to the biological system in which they reside. Association study results were considered significant (sig.) and included in the 'No. sig.' column if the association was significant at $p < 0.05$. No. conducted = total number of studies conducted. BITE = Bulimia Investigation Test Edinburgh; BMI = body mass index; BPD = borderline personality disorder; EAT = Eating Attitudes Test; OCD, obsessive-compulsive disorder.

'Quantitative traits' denotes results from studies that examined associations between genes and levels of disordered eating or other psychopathological behaviors. Studies included in 'Quantitative traits' were also included in the 'Case–control/association studies' totals if both association (i.e. case–control or within-family) *and* quantitative trait analyses were conducted.

aThe quantitative trait was examined in a combined sample of AN or BN, and the results are therefore listed in the columns for both AN and BN studies.

bAssociated with AN-R only.

cAssociated with AN and AN-R.

*Trend $p < 0.10$.

findings are confirming a role for the serotonin 2a receptor and serotonin transporter gene in the etiology of EDs.

Serotonin 2a receptor (5-HT$_{2a}$)

The A allele of the -1438A/G polymorphism of the 5-HT$_{2a}$ gene has been identified previously as a potential risk allele for AN, particularly AN restrictive subtype (AN-R) (see Gorwood et al. 2003; Klump and Gobrogge 2005). Findings for BN have been more equivocal, as studies have reported no significant associations, associations with the A allele, and associations with the G allele (for a review, see Klump and Culbert 2007). Two recent studies found a trend-level association between the A allele and AN (Rybawoski et al. 2006), yet no significant associations were found between the A or G allele and BN (Bruce et al. 2005). Overall, these findings corroborate previous results and suggest that the A allele may contribute to the genetic diathesis of AN.

Studies incorporating quantitative traits have found the A allele to be associated with lower caloric intake and fat consumption in healthy males and females (Herbeth et al. 2005). This allele may therefore be linked to the decreased food intake observed in patients with AN. Patients with AN who were homozygous for the A allele also showed significantly lower levels of reward dependence and harm avoidance than patients with one or two copies of the G allele (Rybawoski et al. 2006). This last set of findings is difficult to interpret, given that higher levels of these traits have been linked to AN (Cassin and von Ranson 2005). The results suggest that within populations of patients with AN, differences in phenotypic characteristics likely reflect genotypic differences in putative risk genes.

Differences in phenotypic traits by genotype have also been observed in BN. Women with BN who were homozygous for the G allele showed significantly increased impulsivity and decreased post-synaptic serotonin activity compared with control women and BN women with at least one copy of the A allele (Bruce et al. 2005). Similar links between the G allele and impulsivity in BN have been reported previously (Nishiguchi et al. 2001), although the opposite pattern of results (i.e. associations between impulsivity and the A allele) was observed in healthy adults (Nomura et al. 2006). Bruce et al. (2005) have proposed that associations between the G allele and increased impulsivity in women with BN may represent characteristics of the illness that are 'activated' by symptoms of BN (i.e. binge eating and vomiting). This hypothesis reconciles inconsistent findings, but should be investigated further before conclusions are drawn.

Taken together, the -1438 A/G polymorphism of the 5-HT$_{2a}$ gene appears to contribute to susceptibility to AN. These findings corroborate previous results, including those from a meta-analysis (Gorwood et al. 2003). This polymorphism may also influence the phenotypic variations (e.g. levels of impulsivity) observed within AN and BN populations (Thompson-Brenner and Westen 2005).

Serotonin transporter (5-HTTLPR/SLC6A4)

Previous studies have reported significant associations between the short ('S') allele of the 5-HTTLPR polymorphism and both AN and BN (Mazzeo et al. 2006), although non-replications have also been reported (e.g., Lauzurica et al. 2003). In the past two years, four studies have examined this polymorphism for EDs, again with mixed results. The findings unexpectedly indicated a higher frequency of the long ('L') allele in patients with BN (Monteleone et al. 2006a) and BED (Monteleone et al. 2006b), and no significant associations between the gene and AN (Rybawoski et al. 2006). However, Urwin and Nunn (2005) found an interaction between the L variant of the monoamine oxidase type A (MAOA) gene and the 5-HTTLPR S/S genotype for AN. Women with both the MAOA L variant and the 5-HTTLPR S/S genotype were at increased risk for AN compared with women who had just one of the gene variants (Urwin and Nunn 2005).

Although the 5-HTTLPR gene may not show <u>direct</u> associations with EDs, it may be linked to phenotypic variations within the disorders. The 'S' allele was linked to higher levels of drive for thinness and body dissatisfaction in patients with AN and BN, suggesting a possible link between the 'S' variant and disorder severity (Frieling et al. 2006). In addition, patients with BN who had at least one copy of the 'S' allele displayed *higher* levels of harm avoidance (Monteleone et al. 2006a), anxiety (Ribasés et al. 2006), affective instability, behavioral impulsivity and comorbid borderline personality disorder (Steiger et al. 2005). Although these findings await replication (for a non-replication using different methods, see Wonderlich et al. 2005), the 'S' allele has been linked to higher levels of serotonin neurotransmission (Steiger et al. 2005), which is implicated in the regulation of mood states (Jimerson and Wolfe 2006). These novel findings suggest that the 'S' allele of 5-HTTLPR is involved in both phenotypic characteristics (e.g. affective dsyregulation, impulsivity) and neurobiological systems (i.e. serotonin) that have been implicated in the development of BN. Thus the 'S' allele of 5-HTTLPR may increase vulnerability to BN via its role in these key features.

Brain-derived neurotrophic factor (BDNF) candidate genes

Research suggests a role for BDNF in the modulation of food intake. Increased BDNF levels have been linked to appetite suppression and weight loss, and decreased levels have been linked to weight gain and obesity (Hashimoto et al. 2005). The primary BDNF gene studied for EDs has been the Val66Met polymorphism. This polymorphism has generally not been associated with either BN (Friedel et al. 2005; Ribasés et al. 2005; Monteleone et al. 2006c) or BED (Monteleone et al. 2006c). However, associations between this polymorphism and AN (particularly AN-R) have been reported previously (Mazzeo et al. 2006). Consistent with these findings, Ribasés et al. (2005) reported a positive association between the Met66 allele and AN-R, as well as excess transmission of the -270C/Met66 haplotype to AN-R probands. Importantly, this study utilized a large sample (n = 359 AN trios) drawn from eight European countries, which increases confidence in the results. However, three other studies found no significant associations between the Val66Met genotype or allele frequencies and AN (de Krom *et al.* 2005; Friedel *et al.* 2005; Dardennes *et al.* 2007). These studies had smaller samples (n = 114–195) and generally did not examine AN-R separately (for an exception, see Dardennes *et al.* 2007).

Interestingly, the Met66 allele and Met-Met genotype were significantly associated with severity of illness (Dardennes *et al.* 2007) and low BMI in individuals with AN-R (Ribasés *et al.* 2005) and a sample of healthy adults (Gunstad *et al.* 2006). The Met66 allele was also significantly associated with AN severity. Taken together, these findings suggest that the Met66 allele may be specifically linked to AN-R and its phenotypic features, such as low body weight.

Conclusions and future directions

Findings from twin studies have continued to indicate a significant role for genes in the etiology of EDs. Consistent with the previous review by Mazzeo *et al.* (2006), the results suggest that:

- genetic influences on certain types of disordered eating symptoms may be gender-differentiated and linked to anxiety
- the serotonin and BDNF systems are promising candidates for genetic influences on EDs
- quantitative traits are valuable additions to molecular genetic analyses.

Importantly, however, new data suggest several additional conclusions that can be drawn.

First, we have more consistent data linking candidate genes to AN (particularly AN-R) than to BN. The -1438 polymorphism of the $5HT_{2a}$ receptor gene and the ValMet66 polymorphism of the BDNF gene are very interesting candidates in this regard. Both of these genes have been linked to AN-R and characteristics associated with the disorder (e.g. low BMI). Both systems are also sexually differentiated and have been associated with anxious traits (Ren-Patterson *et al.* 2006). Based on these data, we cautiously conclude that these genes are likely to be important for the genetic diathesis of AN and may influence genetic risk through food intake, body weight regulation and/or anxious traits.

By contrast, we have less consistent data linking candidate genes to BN. Studies that do find associations tend to find them with phenotypic variations within the disorder rather than with the disorder itself. Indeed, convergent data suggest that the 5-HTTLPR 'S' allele is associated with the affective dysregulation that is present in many women with BN.

These findings highlight critical issues raised previously about phenotypic heterogeneity within BN (Thompson-Brenner and Westen 2005; Wonderlich *et al.* 2005; Klump and Culbert 2007). It is perhaps no coincidence that linkage

(Grice *et al.* 2002) and association studies have been more successful in identifying genes for AN-R, as BN is more heterogeneous in personality and affective profiles (Thompson-Brenner and Westen 2005) than AN or AN-R. Our failure to consistently identify genes for BN may therefore be due to hetero-geneous patient samples that differ in phenotypic *and* genotypic characteristics.

These findings have significant implications for future research. We should continue to narrow phenotypes for analysis, particularly for BN. It will be important to use quantitative traits in these analyses, but also to subtype BN women, similar to what has been done for AN-R. For example, comparing allele and genotype frequencies between women with BN who are multi-impulsive and healthy controls may highlight genes that contribute to the risk for this subtype of BN (for an example of subtyping women with BN in a genetic study, see Wonderlich *et al.* 2005). Subtyping women with BN will advance knowledge beyond understanding genetic contributions to phenotypic variations *within* the disorder to identifying genes that contribute to the etiology of subtypes of the disorder.

Implicit in the above discussion is the recognition that some of the genetic diathesis of AN and BN is likely to be distinct. Linkage study data corroborate this impression, as do candidate gene studies that have generally failed to find genes jointly associated with both disorders. Future studies should continue to examine the extent to which the genes for AN and BN are distinct.

Other fruitful areas for future research include improving upon methodolo-gical limitations and elucidating the nature of genetic effects. Larger samples continue to be needed for all types of genetic research. These samples could be maximized with multi-site collaborations (e.g. Ribasés *et al.* 2005). Researchers should also examine more than one polymorphism per gene in order to determine whether a gene (rather than just a single polymorphism) is associated with EDs. Within these investigations, it will be important to examine gene x gene interactions in effects, as the influence of genes may not be additive. Although investigators have only recently begun to examine these types of interactions, initial evidence suggests that this is a promising area for future research (e.g. Urwin and Nunn 2005). However, genes interact not only with each other, but also with environmental risk factors (Moffitt *et al.* 2005). Future studies should also aim to investigate environmental risk factors (e.g. stressful life events) that may modify genetic risk for EDs. As others have noted (Moffitt *et al.* 2005), non-replications in association studies may be the result of gene x environment interactions in which genes only contribute to EDs in individuals who are exposed to putative environmental risk factors. In addition, if epigen-etic mechanisms are present, in which environmental factors act to change gene expression, non-significant results in candidate gene studies may also be due to these effects. Specifically, alterations of gene function and expression via epigenetic mechanisms (e.g. nutrition) could influence the activation and/or deactivation of genes and modify risk for EDs (see Van den Veyver 2002). Indeed, DNA methylation patterns and histone proteins have been shown to be modified by diet and likely play a role in genomic stability and functioning (Van den Veyver 2002). Efforts aimed at examining the role of epigenetic effects, rather than merely genotypic variation, may improve our understanding of individual differences in genetic effects on risk and expression of eating pathology.

Finally, the genetic basis of EDs may be advanced by elucidating the functional significance of genes and examining endophenotypes. The functional significance of most genes remains unknown, leading to ambiguity about the mechanisms of genetic effects. Moreover, studies would benefit from identifying and incorporating endophenotypes into analyses. Endophenotypes are heritable traits associated with the disorder that are purported to be linked to a smaller number of genes than the disorder itself (for a review of endophenotypes in EDs, see Bulik *et al.* in press). Recent evidence suggests that cognitive set-shifting (Holliday *et al.* 2005) and serotonergic dysfunction (Steiger *et al.* 2006) may be endophenotypes that are involved in the genetic diathesis of EDs. Future research should incorporate these traits into molecular genetic analyses and aim to identify additional endophenotypes for EDs.

Clinical implications

The findings that have been reviewed here have several clinical implications. Perhaps most importantly, clinicians can use this information to reduce parental guilt generated by the view that parents cause EDs in their children. Within this context, it will be important for clinicians to emphasize that genetic risk involves a complex interaction of genetic and environmental factors, and consequently genetic 'risk' for an ED does not imply genetic 'determination' (Mazzeo *et al.* 2006).

Genetic studies may also prove useful for equalizing insurance reimbursement across psychiatric conditions. Treatment for EDs is restricted under many insurance plans in the USA because the conditions are not considered to be 'biologically based'. However, the data strongly suggest that the heritability of EDs (> 50%) (see Bulik *et al.* 2000) is on a par with other disorders that are considered to be biologically based (e.g. schizophrenia and bipolar disorder). Thus the disparity in insurance reimbursement for eating disorders treatment in the USA is without evidential basis and should be discontinued.

Genetic research may also help with treatment and prevention programs. The identification of genes that confer risk for EDs may help in designing pharmacological treatments (Mazzeo *et al.* 2006). Preventive efforts can also be improved by incorporating knowledge of genetic and environmental risk factors into interventions (Mazzeo *et al.* 2006). For example, individuals in the population who are at increased risk, due to family history of eating disorders and related phenotypes, can be identified and targeted for intensive prevention programs.

References

(References included from the targeted review years are preceded by one asterisk. References preceded by three asterisks are of particular significance. The significance is explained by a short commentary following the complete reference.)

***Bacanu S, Bulik C, Klump K, Fichter M, Halmi K, Keel P *et al.* (2005) Linkage analysis of anorexia and bulimia nervosa cohorts using selected behavioral phenotypes as quantitative traits or covariates. *American Journal of Medical Genetics Part B (Neuropsychiatric Genetics),* **139B:** 61–8.

Incorporating quantitative traits (e.g. obsessionality, age at menarche, lowest lifetime BMI) into analyses, this linkage study confirmed previous evidence that regions on chromosomes 1, 4, 10, 11, 13 and 14 may be important for eating disorders. Furthermore, distinct linkage signals were observed for AN and BN, indicating that at least some unique genetic effects underlie these eating disorders.

*Bruce K, Steiger H, Joober R, Ng Ying Kin N, Israel M and Young S (2005) Association of the promoter polymorphism -1438 G/A of the 5-HT2A receptor gene with behavioral impulsiveness and serotonin function in women with bulimia nervosa. *American Journal of Medical Genetics Part B (Neuropsychiatric Genetics),* **137B:** 40–44.

Bulik CM, Sullivan PF and Kendler KS (1998) Heritability of binge-eating and broadly defined bulimia nervosa. *Biological Psychiatry,* **44:** 1210–18.

Bulik CM, Sullivan PF, Wade TD and Kendler KS (2000) Twin studies of eating disorders: a review. *International Journal of Eating Disorders,* **27:** 1–20.

Bulik CM, Wade TD and Kendler KS (2001) Characteristics of monozygotic twins discordant for bulimia nervosa. *International Journal of Eating Disorders,* **29:** 1–10.

Bulik CM, Devlin B, Bacanu SA, Thornton L, Klump KL, Fichter MM *et al.* (2003) Significant linkage on chromosome 10p in families with bulimia nervosa. *American Journal of Human Genetics,* **72:** 200–207.

*Bulik CM, Bacanu SA, Klump KL, Fichter MM, Halmi KA, Keel P *et al.* (2005) Selection of eating-disorder phenotypes for linkage analysis. *American Journal of Medical Genetics Part B (Neuropsychiatric Genetics),* **139B:** 81–7.

*Bulik CM, Hebebrand J, Keski-Rahkonen A, Klump KL, Reichborn-Kjennerud T,

Mazzeo SE *et al.* (in press) Genetic epidemiology, endophenotypes, and eating disorder classification. *International Journal of Eating Disorders..*

*Cassin SE and von Ranson KM (2005) Personality and eating disorders: a decade in review. *Clinical Psychology Review,* **25:** 895–916.

*Dardennes RM, Zizzari P, Tolle V, Foulon C, Kipman A, Romo L *et al.* (2007) Family trios analysis of common polymorphisms in the obestatin/ghrelin, BDNF and AGRP genes in AN: association with subtype, BMI, severity and age of onset. *Psychoneuroendocrinology,* **32:** 106–13.

de Castro JM (1999) Heritability of hunger relationships with food intake in free-living humans. *Physiology and Behavior,* **67:** 249–58.

*de Castro JM and Lilenfeld LRR (2005) Influence of heredity on dietary restraint, disinhibition and perceived hunger in humans. *Nutrition,* **21:** 446–55.

*de Krom M, Bakker S, Hendriks J, van Elburg A, Hoogendoorn M, Verduijn W *et al.*

(2005) Polymorphisms in the brain-derived neurotrophic factor gene are not associated with either anorexia nervosa or schizophrenia in Dutch patients. *Psychiatric Genetics,* **15:** 81.

*Friedel S, Fontenla Horro F, Wermter A, Geller F, Dempfle A, Reichwald K *et al.* (2005) Mutation screen of the brain-derived neurotrophic factor gene (BDNF): identification of

several genetic variants and association studies in patients with obesity, eating disorders, and attention-deficit/hyperactivity disorder. *American Journal of Medical Genetics
Part B (Neuropsychiatric Genetics)*, **132B:** 96–9.

*Frieling H, Romer K, Wilhelm J, Hillemacher T, Kornhuber J, de Zwaan M *et al.* (2006)
Association of catecholamine-O-methyltransferase and 5-HTTLPR genotype with eat-
ing-disorder-related behavior and attitudes in females with eating disorders. *Psychiatric
Genetics*, **16:** 205–8.

Gorwood P, Kipman A and Foulon C (2003) The human genetics of anorexia nervosa.
European Journal of Pharmacology, **480:** 163–70.

Grice DE, Halmi MM, Fichter M, Strober DB, Woodside JT, Treasure AS *et al.* (2002)
Evidence for a susceptibility gene for anorexia nervosa on chromosome 1. *American
Journal of Human Genetics*, **70:** 787–92.

*Gunstad J, Schofield P, Paul RH, Spitznagel MB, Cohen RA, Williams LM *et al.* (2006)
BDNF Val66Met polymorphism is associated with body mass index in healthy adults.
Neuropsychobiology, **53:** 153–6.

*Hashimoto K, Koizumi H, Nakazato M, Shimizu E and Iyo M (2005) Role of brain-derived
neurotrophic factor in eating disorders: recent findings and its pathophysiological
implications. *Progress in Neuro-Psychopharmacology and Biological Psychiatry*, **29:** 499–504.

*Herbeth B, Aubry E, Fumeron F, Aubert R, Cailotto F *et al.* (2005) Polymorphism of the
5HT2A receptor gene and food intake in children and adolescents: the Stanislas Family
Study. *American Journal of Clinical Nutrition*, **82:** 467–70.

*Holliday J, Tchanturia K, Landau S, Collier D and Treasure J (2005) Is impaired set-shifting
an edonphenotype of anorexia nervosa? *American Journal of Psychiatry*, **162:** 2269–75.

*Jimerson DC and Wolfe BE (2006) Psychobiology of eating disorders. In: Wonderlich S,
Mitchell JE, de Zwann M and Steiger H, editors. *Eating Disorders Review. Part 2.* Oxford:
Radcliffe Publishing, pp. 1–16.

*Keel PK, Klump KL, Miller KB, McGue M and Iacono WG (2005) Shared transmission of
eating disorders and anxiety disorders. *International Journal of Eating Disorders*, **38:** 99–
105.

*Keski-Rahkonen A, Neale BM, Bulik CM, Pietilainen KH, Rose RJ Kaprio J *et al.* (2005)
Intentional weight loss in young adults: sex-specific genetic and environmental effects.
Obesity Research, **13:** 745–53.

*Klump KL and Gobrogge KL (2005) A review and primer of molecular genetic studies of
AN. *International Journal of Eating Disorders*, **37:** S43–8.

*Klump KL and Culbert KM (2007) Molecular genetic studies of eating disorders: current
status and future directions. *Current Directions in Psychological Science*, **16:** 37–41.

Lauzurica N, Hurtado A, Escarti A, Delgado M, Barrios V, Morande G *et al.* (2003)
Polymorphisms within the promoter and the intron 2 of the serotonin transporter
gene in a population of bulimic patients. *Neuroscience Letters*, **352:** 226–30.

*Mazzeo SE, Slof-Op't Landt MCT, van Furth EF and Bulik CM (2006) Genetics of eating
disorders. In: Wonderlich S, Mitchell JE, de Zwann M and Steiger H, editors. *Eating
Disorders Review. Part 2.* Oxford: Radcliffe Publishing, pp. 17–33.

*Moffitt TE, Caspi A and Rutter M (2005) Strategy for investigating interactions between
measured genes and measured environments. *Archives of General Psychiatry*, **62:** 473–81.

*Monteleone P, Santonastaso P, Mauro M, Bellodi L, Erzegovesi S, Fuschino A *et al.* (2006a)
Investigation of the serotonin transporter regulatory region polymorphism in bulimia
nervosa: relationships to harm avoidance, nutritional parameters, and psychiatric
comorbidity. *Psychosomatic Medicine*, **68:** 99–103.

*Monteleone P, Tortella A, Castaldo E and Maj M (2006b) Association of a functional
serotonin transporter gene polymorphism with binge-eating disorder. *American Journal
of Medical Genetics Part B (Neuropsychiatric Genetics)*, **141B:** 7–9.

*Monteleone P, Zanardini R, Tortorella A, Gennarelli M, Castaldo E, Canestrelli B *et al.* (2006c) The 196G/A (val66met) polymorphism of the BDNF gene is significantly associated with binge eating behavior in women with bulimia nervosa or binge eating disorder. *Neuroscience Letters*, **406**: 133–7.

Nishiguchi N, Matsuchita S, Suzuki K, Murayama M, Shirakawa O and Higuchi S (2001) Association between 5HT2A receptor gene promoter region polymorphism and eating disorders in Japanese patients. *Biological Psychiatry*, **15**: 123–8.

*Nomura M, Kusumi I, Kaneko M, Masui T, Daiguji M, Ueno T *et al.* (2006) Involvement of a polymorphism in the 5-HT2A receptor gene in impulsive behavior. *Psychopharmacology*, **187**: 30–35.

*Ren-Patterson R, Cochran LW, Holmes A, Lesch KP, Lu B and Murphy DL (2006) Gender-dependent modulation of brain monoamines and anxiety-like behaviors in mice with genetic serotonin transporter and BDNF deficiencies. *Cellular and Molecular Neurobiology*, **26**: 753–78.

***Ribasés M, Gratacòs M, Fernández-Aranda F, Bellodi L, Boni C, Anderluh M *et al.* (2005) Association of BDNF with restricting anorexia nervosa and minimum body mass index: a family-based association study of eight European populations. *European Journal of Human Genetics*, **13**: 428–34.

This study examined associations between the Val66Met and -270C/T polymorphisms of the BDNF gene, AN, BN and phenotypic traits (e.g. BMI). Notably, a large sample of family trios from a multi-site collaboration were obtained for analyses. The findings supported a role for the Met66 variant in both AN-R and minimum BMI.

*Ribasés M, Fernandez-Aranda F, Gratacòs M, Mercader JM, Casasnovas C, Núñez A *et al.* (in press) Contribution of the serotonergic system to anxious and depressive traits that may be partially responsible for the phenotypical variability of bulimia nervosa. *Journal of Psychiatric Research*.

*Rybawoski F, Slopien A, Dmitrzak-Weglarz M, Czerski P, Rajwski A and Hauser J (2006) The 5-HT2A -1438 A/G and 5-HTTLPR polymorphisms and personality dimensions in adolescent anorexia nervosa: association study. *Neuropsychobiology*, **53**: 33–9.

***Steiger H, Joober R, Israel M, Young SN, Ng Ying Kin N, Gauvin L *et al.* (2005) The 5-HTTLPR polymorphism, psychopathologic symptoms, and platelet [^{3}H-] paroxetine binding in bulimic syndromes. *International Journal of Eating Disorders*, **37**: 57–60.

Using a multi-method approach, significant associations were found between the "S" variant of the 5-HTTLPR polymorphism and mood and behavioral symptoms (e.g. affective instability, impulsivity). Importantly, associations were also observed with reduced serotonin reuptake in the periphery, as evidenced by reduced platelet [3H-] paroxetine binding. Thus, vulnerability to various characteristics that have been implicated in the development of BN may be codetermined by the "S" variant.

***Steiger H, Gauvin L, Joober R, Israel M, Ng Ying Kin NMK, Bruce KR *et al.* (2006) Intrafamilial correspondences on platelet [^{3}H-] paroxetine binding in bulimic probands and their unaffected first-degree relatives. *Neuropsychopharmacology*, **31**: 1785–92.

This investigation indicated that 5-HT transporter activity may be an endophenotype involved in the genetic diathesis of BN. Specifically, unaffected female relatives of women with BN displayed significantly lower 5-HT transporter activity than control women, yet similar 5-HT transporter activity to that of their affected BN relative.

*Tholin S, Rasmussen F, Tynelius P and Karlsson J (2005) Genetic and environmental influences on eating behavior: the Swedish Young Male Twins Study. *American Journal of Clinical Nutrition*, **81**: 564–9.

*Thompson-Brenner H and Westen D (2005) Personality subtypes in eating disorders: validation of a classification in a naturalistic sample. *British Journal of Psychiatry*, **186**: 516–24.

***Urwin R and Nunn K (2005) Epistatic interaction between the monoamine oxidase A and serotonin transporter genes in anorexia nervosa. *European Journal of Human Genetics*, **13:** 370–75.

This study examined whether the S/S genotype of the 5-HTTLPR polymorphism and L-variant of the MAOA gene interact in the risk for AN. It was found that risk for AN was eight times greater in women with both the MAOA L variant and the S/S genotype than in women with the MAOA-L variant alone.

Van den Veyver IB (2002) Genetic effects of methylation diets. *Annual Review of Nutrition*, **22:** 255–82.

*Wonderlich SA, Crosby RD, Joiner T, Peterson CB, Bardone-Cone A, Klein M *et al.* (2005) Personality subtyping and bulimia nervosa: psychopathological and genetic correlates. *Psychological Medicine*, **35:** 649–57.

3

Sociocultural influences on eating disorders

Pamela K Keel and Julie A Gravener

Abstract

Objectives of review. This chapter reviews articles published in 2005 and 2006 on the influence of culture, ethnicity and gender on eating disorders. Specific social environmental factors, including media portrayals of body ideals and peer and family environment, are also reviewed.

Summary of recent findings. Certain non-Western values may increase the risk of eating disorders. Ethnicity and gender may moderate associations between risk factors and disordered eating. The media promote different body image ideals for women and men that may contribute to gender differences in the rates and expression of eating disorders. Peers and family translate broad cultural values into personally relevant ideals that influence behavior.

Future directions. Much of the research on sociocultural factors remains focused on the role of the thin ideal. Future work could examine the influence of collectivism, anonymity, and shifts from multigenerational to predominantly peer social environments as possible sociocultural factors that increase the risk of eating disorders.

Introduction

Eating disorders are most likely to occur in females from industrialized nations (American Psychiatric Association 2000), and appear to be less common among some ethnic subgroups (Striegel-Moore *et al.* 2003). These patterns raise questions about how membership of a given culture, ethnic group and gender influence disordered eating. We review literature that addresses cultural influences on eating disorders. In addition, we examine how social factors, such as peer and family environment, influence risk. We view social and cultural factors as representing levels of influence. However, the organization of this review is not meant to imply a unidirectional order of influence. For example, gender is negotiated within cultural and ethnic groups, yet certain aspects of gender may transcend cultural or ethnic group boundaries (Safir *et al.* 2005).

Studies were identified through electronic searches of MEDLINE and Psy-chINFO using 13 eating-related terms (e.g. eating disorders, anorexia nervosa, bulimia nervosa) and 19 sociocultural terms (e.g. culture, ethnicity, family) for articles published in English between 2005 and 2006. A total of 166 articles were considered for inclusion. Primary reasons for exclusion were article topic and methodology. We identified certain themes for each section, and articles that did not address these themes or include key measures or analyses were excluded.

Cross-cultural comparisons

Previous work has demonstrated cross-cultural differences in the presence of eating disorders (Keel and Klump 2003). The impact of Western ideals and rapid cultural transitions on disordered eating has been the focus of previous work (Becker and Fay 2006). Articles published in 2005 and 2006 have continued this tradition (Stark-Wroblewski *et al.* 2005; Eapen *et al.* 2006; Williams *et al.* 2006), but have extended examination of cross-cultural differences to look beyond the 'Westernization hypothesis' (Soh *et al.* 2006). A new generation of studies has focused on non-Western cultural ideals that may either protect against (Hoek *et al.* 2005) or increase risk for eating disorders (Jackson *et al.* 2006).

Hoek and colleagues (Hoek *et al.* 2005) examined the incidence of anorexia nervosa (AN) in Curacao, a Caribbean island with a predominantly black population. This study is noteworthy because of its thorough ascertainment and assessment of cases. AN incidence differed markedly by ethnic subgroup. No cases were detected among the majority black population, whereas AN incidence in white and mixed-race populations was similar to rates observed in the USA and the Netherlands. The authors posited that sociocultural factors explained these dramatic differences. All individuals with AN had been abroad for at least a year, and most (64%) had been abroad before the onset of AN. Although Dutch and US television was described as 'widely available', the authors noted that being overweight is more socially acceptable among the African-Caribbean population of Curacao. Thus, despite rapid cultural transition, black women in Curacao may be protected from developing AN by traditional values that embrace a larger body ideal.

In contrast to the results of Hoek and colleagues (Hoek *et al.* 2005), several articles have posited risk factors for the development of eating disorders that are native to Asian cultures, including Korea (Jackson *et al.* 2006), Thailand (Jennings *et al.* 2006) and Japan (Kusano-Scharz and von Wietersheim 2005). Wardle *et al.* (2006) examined self-reported height and weight, perceived weight, and attempts to lose weight using a self-report survey in 18,512 college students administered in 22 countries in their native languages. Perceptions of weight and attempts to lose weight were plotted against population-specific BMI norms to control for regional differences. Perceptions of overweight and attempts to lose weight were highest in Asian countries (Korea, Thailand and Japan), lowest in Mediterranean countries (Greece, Italy, Portugal and Spain), and moderate both in North-West Europe (Belgium, UK, France, Germany, Iceland, Ireland and the Netherlands) and the USA, and in the former socialist states of Central and Eastern Europe (Bulgaria, Hungary, Poland, Romania and Slovakia). The authors commented that "Contrary to our expectations, women in the USA and UK reported moderate levels of weight concern, while women from Asia reported extremely high levels" (p. 650). However, these results are largely consistent with a growing body of literature which suggests that the incidence of disordered eating may be elevated in Asian countries compared with Western countries.

Jackson *et al.* (2006) compared disordered eating in three groups of Korean women, namely Korean women in Korea (native Koreans), Korean immigrants in the USA, and second-generation Korean Americans. The incidence of disordered eating was higher in the native Korean and Korean immigrant groups than in the Korean American group. Furthermore, a measure of acculturation demonstrated no association with levels of disordered eating in the two US samples. These results failed to support the Westernization hypothesis, as the group with the greatest immersion in Western ideals and culture (Korean Americans) had the least eating pathology. Similarly, higher rates of disordered eating have been reported in Thai women in Thailand compared with both Asian and Caucasian women in Australia (Jennings *et al.* 2006), and higher rates have been reported in women and BN patients in Japan compared with their counterparts in Germany (Kusano-Scharz and von Wietersheim 2005).

Authors who have found an elevated incidence of disordered eating in Asian countries have discussed several aspects of Asian cultures that may influence risk. In Korea, Confucian-based gender roles define women's value primarily by their ability to marry into prominent families, and modern-day matchmakers in Korea (*kyol honsangdam-so*) rate women most highly on physical appearance, consistent with a cultural emphasis on appearance over ability for women (Jackson *et al.* 2006). Similarly, Thai culture emphasizes the importance of women's beauty for holding men's attention and maintaining status (Jennings *et al.* 2006). Thus the combination of importing the Western thin ideal and gender roles that emphasize physical appearance as defining women's value may contribute to the particularly high risk of developing eating disorders in Korean and Thai cultures. In addition, authors have noted the potential influence of collectivism on the development of disordered eating in Asian cultures (Kusano-Scharz and von Wietersheim 2005; Jackson *et al.* 2006; Jennings *et al.* 2006). Collectivism emphasizes the needs and desires of the group over those of the individual, in contrast to individualism, which emphasizes autonomy and the needs and desires of the individual. Kusano-Schwartz and von Wiestersheim (2005) described Japanese culture as emphasizing "harmony with the values of society", and speculated that the higher levels of disordered eating in Japan may reflect greater penetration of unhealthy ideals in a culture that equates self-realization with the realization of social values (p. 415).

Cummins *et al.* (2005) suggested several additional factors for an exploration of Asian culture's contribution to eating disorder development, including cultural attitudes towards eating, control, and regulation of emotion. The authors argue that such culturally informed factors may mediate associations between identified risk factors and disordered eating. Of interest, it has been found that body dissatisfaction mediated the association between self-esteem and disordered eating in Australian women but not in Hong Kong women. Instead, self-esteem mediated the association between body dissatisfaction and disordered eating in Hong Kong women (Sheffield *et al.* 2005). Although these models were based on cross-sectional data and thus do not test causal mediation models, they provide insights into potential cultural differences in developmental pathways for disordered eating.

Ethnicity

A recent review (Grabe and Hyde 2006) documented a preponderance of studies comparing white and black population samples with other ethnic subgroups with regard to body image. However, most of the studies that we reviewed compared multiple ethnic groups. This provides a rich resource for understanding how subgroups within a culture may differ with regard to body image and disordered eating. The following section reviews such differences, and evidence is then presented that ethnicity may moderate associations between risk factors and disordered eating.

In a meta-analysis of 222 effect sizes from 98 studies, Grabe and Hyde (2006) found small but significant differences in African-American compared with Caucasian and Hispanic females, with African-American individuals reporting less body dissatisfaction. Consistent with these results, eating disorder symptoms were found to be lower in African-American and Caribbean girls compared with Hispanic and non-Hispanic white girls (Bisaga *et al.* 2005), and black college women reported less dieting than white college women (Aruguete *et al.* 2005; York-Crowe and Williamson 2005). Furthermore, a study conducted in South Africa (le Grange *et al.* 2006) reported higher Eating Attitude Test-26 scores in white adolescent females compared with their black African and mixed race counterparts. However, no racial differences were found in adult women or males (le Grange *et al.* 2006). In addition, scores on the Bulimia Investigatory Test, Edinburgh (BITE) were higher in black African women and males than in their white and mixed race counterparts (le Grange *et al.* 2006). These results suggest that the effects of race may differ substantially between the USA and South Africa. However, some US studies have not found significant differences in disordered eating between black or African-American participants and Caucasian groups (Reagan and Hersch 2005; Cachelin and Regan 2006) or Hispanic groups (Cachelin and Regan 2006; Regan and Cachelin 2006). Moreover, the results are consistent with findings from recent meta-analytic studies in suggesting that stereotypic effects (e.g. white populations having higher levels of disordered eating than black populations) may only be evident in older adolescent groups (Grabe and Hyde 2006; Roberts *et al.* 2006), that different measures produce different results (Grabe and Hyde 2006), and that less robust differences have been found in more recent studies (Grabe and Hyde 2006; Roberts *et al.* 2006).

Grabe and Hyde (2006) did not find meaningful differences in body dissatisfaction among Hispanic, Asian and Caucasian women in their meta-analysis. Again these results are consistent with comparisons of disordered eating levels in high school girls (Bisaga *et al.* 2005). Similarly, few differences were found between Hispanic and Caucasian females in community-based studies of dieting (Cachelin and Regan 2006) and disordered eating (Regan and Cachelin 2006). Higher socioeconomic status (SES) (Granillo *et al.* 2005) and greater Anglo acculturation (Cachelin *et al.* 2006a) have been associated with more disordered eating in Latinas.

Despite evidence of similar levels of body dissatisfaction in Asian and Caucasian women (Cummins *et al.* 2005; Grabe and Hyde 2006), studies have reported lower levels of disordered eating in Asian women compared with other ethnic groups (Cachelin and Regan 2006; Regan and Cachelin 2006) in both the USA and the UK (Cummins *et al.* 2005). These patterns led Cummins *et al.* (2005) to question whether certain sociocultural factors might blunt the association between body dissatisfaction and disordered eating in Asian individuals.

As described above, ethnicity may influence eating disorders either by impacting on risk factor levels or by moderating associations between risk factors and disordered eating. In a comprehensive assessment of risk factors for binge-eating disorder (BED) in black and white women in the USA, Striegel-Moore *et al.* (2005) found little evidence that ethnicity moderated associations between risk factors and eating pathology. Similarly, Harrison and Hefner (2006) found no evidence that ethnicity moderated prospective associations between television viewing and disordered eating in adolescent girls. However, Hispanic ethnic identity has been found to moderate associations between awareness and internalization of the thin ideal and between internalization of the thin ideal and body dissatisfaction, such that less robust associations were found in Spanish and Mexican American college students compared with Caucasian college students (Warren *et al.* 2005). Finally, Phan and Tylka (2006) found no evidence that Asian ethnic identity moderated associations between body image variables and eating disorder symptoms in college women.

Gender

Among sociocultural factors that influence eating disorders, gender is perhaps the most influential, as these disorders predominantly affect women. In addition, gender differences have emerged in risk factors for eating pathology (Grilo and Masheb 2005; Hospers and Jansen 2005; Meyer *et al.* 2005) and expression of eating pathology (Weltzin *et al.* 2005; Harrison *et al.* 2006; Varnado-Sullivan *et al.* 2006). Gender differences in the strength of association between body image and self-esteem have received greater attention in the recent literature. Body image disturbance and poor self-esteem have been identified as risk factors for the development of eating disorders, and both are more common in girls than in boys (Elgin and Pritchard 2006). In addition, undue influence of weight or shape on self-evaluation is a defining feature of both AN and BN, according to the DSM-IV. Thus gender differences in a link between body image and self-evaluation could further explain why men are under-represented among those suffering from AN and BN (Elgin and Pritchard 2006). The following section reviews research on the moderating effect of gender on associations between body image and self-esteem.

Davison and McCabe (2006) examined associations between different aspects of body image and self-esteem in a large sample of adolescent girls and boys. The authors found similar associations between body image (broadly defined) and self-esteem between genders. However, for girls, the way in which others might evaluate their body weight and shape was most strongly associated with their self-esteem, whereas for boys, general appearance, facial attractiveness and 'looks' were more strongly associated with self-esteem (Davison and McCabe 2006). In college students, body dissatisfaction was significantly associated with self-esteem in women but not in men (Elgin and Pritchard 2006). Such differences could contribute to gender differences in the extreme weight loss behaviors and increased risk of eating disorders observed in females. However, body image ideals differ between the genders, emphasizing thinness for girls and muscularity for boys. Thus, gender differences in extreme weight loss behaviors may not reflect the strength of the association between body image and self-esteem.

Kashubeck-West et al. (2005) attempted to control for gender differences in desire for weight loss by studying a large sample of men and women who all were attempting to lose weight. Although controlling for desired weight loss eliminated gender differences in overall body dissatisfaction and importance of weight in self-evaluation, the authors found a greater number of significant associations between satisfaction with specific body parts and self-esteem in women compared with men. In addition, women employed more weight loss strategies, such as eating low-calorie foods, eating according to a special diet, and counting calories, compared with men (Kashubeck-West et al. 2005), which suggests that gender differences in associations between self-esteem and body image may be mirrored by gender differences in eating behaviors even after controlling for desire to lose weight.

In a longitudinal study of women and men first assessed in college and then followed for 10 years, McKinley (2006) found that associations between body esteem and self-acceptance diminished over time in women, and no longer differed from the associations found in men at follow-up. Thus, the period of peak risk for eating disorders in women is marked by a moderating effect of gender on associations between body image and self-esteem.

A theme that runs through the above sections is the influence of culture, ethnicity and gender on desire to lose weight. Thus, the sociocultural influence on body image ideals is an important factor to consider. Because body image is covered in a separate section of the *Annual Review* (*see* page 69), we shall only comment briefly on the recent literature that connects media influence on body image ideals in relation to gender differences. Women have been bombarded with media images of the thin ideal for several decades. In recent years, men have received greater attention as a potential market for appearance-related products. Thus, several recent articles have utilized experimental designs to examine the influence of media portrayals of the thin ideal on women versus their portrayals of the muscular ideal on men.

Several papers have documented that exposure to media images of thin models causes increased body dissatisfaction in women (Birkeland *et al.*, 2005; Brown and Dittmar 2005; Clay *et al.* 2005; Bessenoff 2006). Recent research has also documented that exposure to media images of muscular models causes increased body dissatisfaction in men (Arbour and Ginis 2006; Baird and Grieve 2006). Thus, both women and men appear to be vulnerable to media messages concerning body image ideals. However, the consequences of these messages probably differ. Harrison *et al.* (2006) experimentally manipulated exposure to body ideals in women and men in order to examine their impact on food intake in front of same-sex peers. Thin ideal images caused women with discrepant current and ideal figures to consume less food. In contrast, muscular ideal images caused men with discrepant current and ideal figures to consume *more* food in front of same-sex peers. Further support for a link between media influence and disordered eating is provided by a longitudinal study of a large sample of adolescent girls, which found that time spent watching television at baseline predicted increases in disordered eating at one-year follow-up (Harrison and Hefner 2006). Thus, media images directed towards women and men may alter eating behaviors. However, men exhibit behaviors that differ from those typically associated with eating disorders (Cafri *et al.* 2006).

Although media images contribute to the development of eating pathology, most individuals who are exposed to media ideals do not develop eating disorders. Studies have found that the effects of media, peers and families coalesce to create a 'subculture' (Levine *et al.* 1994) that further reinforces cultural body ideals and increases disordered eating (McCabe and Ricciardelli 2005a, 2005b; Muris *et al.* 2005; Smolak *et al.* 2005; Ricciardelli *et al.* 2006). Thus, it is important to examine peer and familial influences as levels closer to the individual that may translate broad social messages into personally relevant risk factors.

Peers

Peer acceptance is of paramount importance during adolescence, and given that acceptance may be contingent upon shared attitudes and behaviors, individuals in this age range may be particularly susceptible to peer influence on disordered eating. Indeed, peer influence has been shown to predict body dissatisfaction (Dohnt and Tiggemann 2005, 2006; McCabe and Ricciardelli 2005a; Paxton *et al.* 2006) and disordered eating in adolescent girls (Shroff and Thompson 2006). Furthermore, perceived friend dieting and school-wide prevalence of dieting were significantly related to engagement in unhealthy weight control behaviors (e.g. diet pill use, purging) among average weight and moderately overweight girls (Eisenberg *et al.* 2005). Thus, girls may equate fitting in with their peers to fitting into a pair of jeans.

Teasing has been examined as a specific mechanism of peer influence, with studies supporting its influence on body image (Eisenberg *et al.* 2006; Lunde *et al.* 2006), body change strategies (Smolak *et al.* 2005) and disordered eating (Muris and Littel 2005). Given the detrimental effects of peer teasing, it is important to identify who is at risk for teasing. Jones and Crawford (2006) found that overweight girls and underweight boys were most likely to be teased about their appearance by peers, which suggests that the immediate social environment plays an important role in enforcing gender-based ideals. However, gender differences may not emerge until adolescence, as a study in 10-year-old children found a significant positive association between BMI and teasing about appearance in both girls and boys (Lunde *et al.* 2006).

Other studies have looked at similarities in eating pathology among groups of friends as an indicator of peer influence. Shroff and Thompson (2006) found no significant correlations among friends on measures of eating pathology in a mid-adolescent sample. However, a longitudinal study of college students found significant peer similarity with regard to bulimic symptoms among friends (Zalta and Keel 2006). Peer similarity was associated with time spent together, and these differences disappeared after an extended separation, which suggests that living among peers may enhance socialization of bulimic symptoms. This could explain the lack of associations found in Shroff and Thompson's high school sample, as most high school students live with and therefore eat several meals per day with their parents.

Utilizing an experimental design, Rotenberg *et al.* (2005) exposed college women to a behaviorally and verbally restrained model, a behaviorally restrained model or no model during an ostensive taste test. The model's dietary restraint impacted on participants' food intake, and the direction of the effect (i.e. increased or decreased intake) depended on individual attribution style for food intake. In a second experimental study, women were exposed to either a confederate conforming to the thin ideal or one of average size (Krones *et al.* 2005). Only women in the thin ideal condition demonstrated increased body dissatisfaction. Thus, experimental studies support causal relationships between peer influence and body image and eating.

Family

Family interactions typically represent a significant proportion of social interactions for children and adolescents. Thus, family members may be an important source of information about eating and body-related behaviors early in life. Supporting this view, more familial influence on weight control was associated with greater internalization of the thin ideal in women (Tester and Gleaves 2005). Familial reinforcement of societal messages may take place through parental modeling of behavior, with studies finding associations between parent and child eating behaviors (Elfhag and Linne 2005; Lamerz *et al.* 2005), dieting (Hirokane *et al.* 2005) and activity levels (Davis *et al.* 2005). Although genes influence associations between parent and child behaviors, behavioral genetic research indicates that shared environment factors explain a significant proportion of variance in disordered eating in young girls (Klump *et al.* 2000).

Beyond modeling, mothers' discussion and encouragement of dieting may reinforce the thin ideal and contribute to dieting and disordered eating in their daughters. Mother–daughter discussions about dieting have been associated with daughters' dieting (Hirokane *et al.* 2005), and maternal encouragement to lose weight has been associated with daughters' dietary restraint (Francis and Birch 2005). Finally, maternal messages regarding weight and shape have been associated with daughters' eating disorder symptoms (Hanna and Bond 2006).

Finally, families may contribute to gender differences in body image ideals and disordered eating. Although significant associations between mother–daughter measures of body dissatisfaction and disordered eating have been found, no significant associations have been found between mothers and sons (Elfhag and Linne 2005). Parental teasing predicted Eating Disorder Inventory drive for thinness and bulimia scores in girls (Keery *et al.* 2005) and muscle-building techniques in adolescent boys (Smolak *et al.* 2005). These results may reflect the extent to which girls perceive their parents as influencing them to lose weight whereas boys perceive their parents as encouraging them to increase their muscularity (McCabe and Ricciardelli 2005b).

Summary of important findings

The studies reviewed above provide strong evidence for the influence of culture, ethnicity, gender, peers and family on disordered eating. These effects appear to be largely mediated by sociocultural influences on body image ideals that are promulgated by the mass media in industrialized nations. However, recent research highlights the potential impact of non-Western values on disordered eating, such as gender roles that emphasize ability to marry into a prominent family, or collectivism. In addition, research has clarified the importance of not approaching ethnic differences as being 'black and white'. Instead, the influence of ethnicity on eating disorders and associations between risk factors and disordered eating depends to a large extent on the ethnic group under investigation. Finally, peers and family members may reinforce cultural body ideals through modeling, discussion and teasing.

Clinical implications

The studies reviewed in this chapter confirm the influence of culture, ethnicity and gender on eating disorders. Although research has largely debunked the stereotype that these are uniquely 'white' female problems, recent work has documented greater barriers to treatment in ethnic minority women compared with white women (Cachelin and Striegel-Moore 2006; Cachelin *et al.* 2006b). Some of this appears to be related to ethnic differences in treatment seeking. However, the evidence suggests that there is decreased recognition of eating disorders when they occur in stereotype-incongruent individuals (Cachelin and Striegel-Moore 2006; Cachelin *et al.* 2006b; Gordon *et al.* 2006). Thus, more work is needed to improve health care professionals' recognition of eating disorders as they occur in diverse groups. In addition, to the extent that factors unrelated to the Western female thin ideal contribute to the development and expression of eating pathology, therapies should examine a wider spectrum of possible sociocultural contributing factors. Finally, interventions, particularly those aimed at preventing eating disorders, may benefit from using peer counselors, given that peers represent a relevant reference group for adolescent behavior.

Future directions

Much of the research on sociocultural factors remains focused on the role of the thin ideal. In addition to the presence of mass media, industrialized nations differ from non-industrialized nations in the presence of urban environments. Importantly, recent work has replicated a link between urbanization and the incidence of BN in the Netherlands (van Son *et al.* 2006). Interestingly, these urban–rural comparisons control for exposure to mass media images, because television, movies and magazines are widely available in both rural and urban regions of Western nations. Thus, the results suggest that the thin ideal may be communicated and reinforced by the immediate social environment, and that factors beyond the pervasiveness of the thin ideal may contribute to eating disorders in industrialized nations. Sociocultural factors that characterize urban environments, such as relative anonymity (van Son *et al.* 2006), access to large stores that stock readily edible foods, and increased contact with same-age peers, may further explain the elevated eating disorder rates in industrialized nations. Put simply, cross-cultural differences in disordered eating may reflect differences in opportunities to engage in symptoms, such as increased time spent alone or with a social group that has more permissive attitudes towards disordered eating. Future research could examine collectivism, anonymity, and shifts from multigenerational to predominantly peer social environments as possible socio-cultural factors that influence the risk of developing eating disorders.

References

(References included from the targeted review years are preceded by one asterisk. References preceded by three asterisks are of particular significance. The significance is explained by a short commentary following the complete reference.)

American Psychiatric Association (2000) *Diagnostic and Statistical Manual of Mental Disorders. Fourth Edition – Text Revision (DSM-IV-TR).* Washington, DC: American Psychiatric Association.

*Arbour KP and Ginis KM (2006) Effects of exposure to muscular and hypermuscular media images on young men's muscularity dissatisfaction and body dissatisfaction. *Body Image*, 3: 153–61.

*Aruguete MS, DeBord KA, Yates A and Edman J (2005) Ethnic and gender differences in eating attitudes among black and white college students. *Eating Behavior*, 6: 328–36.

*Baird AL and Grieve FG (2006) Exposure to male models in advertisements leads to a decrease in men's body satisfaction. *North American Journal of Psychology*, 8: 115–21.

*Becker A and Fay K, editors (2006) *Sociocultural Issues and Eating Disorders*. Oxford: Radcliffe Publishing.

*Bessenoff GR (2006) Can the media affect us? Social comparison, self-discrepancy, and the thin ideal. *Psychology of Women Quarterly*, **30**: 239–51.

*Birkeland R, Thompson JK, Herbozo S, Roehrig M, Cafri G and van den Berg P (2005) Media exposure, mood, and body image dissatisfaction: an experimental test of person versus product priming. *Body Image*, **2**: 53–61.

*Bisaga K, Whitaker A, Davies M, Chuang S, Feldman J and Walsh BT (2005) Eating disorder and depressive symptoms in urban high school girls from different ethnic backgrounds. *Journal of Developmental and Behavioral Pediatrics*, **26**: 257–66.

*Brown A and Dittmar H (2005) Think "thin" and feel bad: the role of appearance schema activation, attention level, and thin-ideal internalization in young women's responses to ultra-thin media ideals. *Journal of Social and Clinical Psychology*, **24**: 1088–113.

*Cachelin FM and Regan PC (2006) Prevalence and correlates of chronic dieting in a multi-ethnic U.S. community sample. *Eating and Weight Disorders*, **11**: 91–9.

***Cachelin FM and Striegel-Moore RH (2006) Help seeking and barriers to treatment in a community sample of Mexican American and European American women with eating disorders. *International Journal of Eating Disorders*, **39**: 154–61.

Although disordered eating does not differ between Hispanic and Caucasian women, Hispanic women are under-represented in studies of eating disorders. This study documents how ethnic differences in treatment seeking and clinician biases may account for this effect.

*Cachelin FM, Phinney JS, Schug RA and Striegel-Moore RM (2006a) Acculturation and eating disorders in a Mexican American community sample. *Psychology of Women Quarterly*, **30**: 340–47.

*Cachelin FM, Striegel-Moore RM and Regan PC (2006b) Factors associated with treatment seeking in a community sample of European American and Mexican American women with eating disorders. *European Eating Disorders Review*, **14**: 422–9.

*Cafri G, van den Berg P and Thompson JK (2006) Pursuit of muscularity in adolescent boys: relations among biopsychosocial variables and clinical outcomes. *Journal of Clinical Child and Adolescent Psychology*, **35**: 283–91.

*Clay D, Vignoles VL and Dittmar H (2005) Body image and self-esteem among adolescent girls: testing the influence of sociocultural factors. *Journal of Research on Adolescence*, **15**: 451–77.

*Cummins LH, Simmons AM and Zane NW (2005) Eating disorders in Asian populations: a critique of current approaches to the study of culture, ethnicity, and eating disorders. *American Journal of Orthopsychiatry*, **75**: 553–74.

*Davis C, Blackmore E, Katzman DK and Fox J (2005) Female adolescents with anorexia nervosa and their parents: a case–control study of exercise attitudes and behaviours. *Psychological Medicine*, **35**: 377–86.

*Davison TE and McCabe MP (2006) Adolescent body image and psychosocial functioning. *Journal of Social Psychology*, **146**: 15–30.

*Dohnt HK and Tiggemann M (2005) Peer influences on body dissatisfaction and dieting awareness in young girls. *British Journal of Developmental Psychology*, **23**: 103–16.

*Dohnt HK and Tiggemann M (2006) Body image concerns in young girls: the role of peers and media prior to adolescence. *Journal of Youth and Adolescence*, **35**: 141–51.

*Eapen V, Mabrouk AA and Bin-Othman S (2006) Disordered eating attitudes and symptomatology among adolescent girls in the United Arab Emirates. *Eating Behavior*, **7**: 53–60.

*Eisenberg ME, Neumark-Sztainer D, Story M and Perry C (2005) The role of social norms and friends' influences on unhealthy weight-control behaviors among adolescent girls. *Social Science and Medicine,* **60:** 1165–73.

*Eisenberg ME, Neumark-Sztainer D, Haines J and Wall M (2006) Weight-teasing and emotional well-being in adolescents: longitudinal findings from Project EAT. *Journal of Adolescent Health,* **38:** 675–83.

*Elfhag K and Linne Y (2005) Gender differences in associations of eating pathology between mothers and their adolescent offspring. *Obesity Research,* **13:** 1070–6.

*Elgin J and Pritchard M (2006) Gender differences in disordered eating and its correlates. *Eating and Weight Disorders,* **11:** 96–101.

*Francis LA and Birch LL (2005) Maternal influences on daughters' restrained eating behavior. *Health Psychology,* **24:** 548–54.

*Gordon KH, Brattole MM, Wingate LR and Joiner TE Jr. (2006) The impact of client race on clinician detection of eating disorders. *Behavior Therapy,* **37:** 319–25.

***Grabe S and Hyde JS (2006) Ethnicity and body dissatisfaction among women in the United States: a meta-analysis. *Psychological Bulletin,* **132:** 622–40.
This comprehensive meta-analysis examined 222 effects sizes from 98 studies. The results debunk the myth that body dissatisfaction is unique to Caucasian women.

*Granillo T, Jones-Rodriguez G and Carvajal SC (2005) Prevalence of eating disorders in Latina adolescents: associations with substance use and other correlates. *Journal of Adolescent Health,* **36:** 214–20.

*Grilo CM and Masheb RM (2005) Correlates of body image dissatisfaction in treatment-seeking men and women with binge eating disorder. *International Journal of Eating Disorders,* **38:** 162–6.

*Hanna AC and Bond MJ (2006) Relationships between family conflict, perceived maternal verbal messages, and daughters' disturbed eating symptomatology. *Appetite,* **47:** 205–11.

*Harrison K and Hefner V (2006) Media exposure, current and future body ideals, and disordered eating among preadolescent girls: a longitudinal panel study. *Journal of Youth and Adolescence,* **35:** 153–63.

***Harrison K, Taylor LD and Marske A (2006) Women's and men's eating behavior following exposure to ideal-body images and text. *Communication Research,* **33:** 507–29.
Utilizing an experimental design, this paper demonstrated how gender differences in body image ideals give rise to gender differences in food intake.

*Hirokane K, Tokumura M, Nanri S, Kimura K and Saito I (2005) Influences of mothers' dieting behaviors on their junior high school daughters. *Eating and Weight Disorders,* **10:** 162–7.

***Hoek HW, van Harten PN, Hermans KM, Katzman MA, Matroos GE and Susser ES (2005) The incidence of anorexia nervosa on Curacao. *American Journal of Psychiatry,* **162:** 748–52.
This study utilized a two-stage design to examine cultural differences in AN incidence. Possible cases were screened for DSM-IV eating disorders after review of hospital records for all inpatients and health care professional screens of outpatient cases from 1995 to 1998. Probable cases underwent structured clinical interviews for eating disorders.

*Hospers HJ and Jansen A (2005) Why homosexuality is a risk factor for eating disorders in males. *Journal of Social and Clinical Psychology,* **24:** 1188–201.

*Jackson SC, Keel PK and Ho Lee Y (2006) Trans-cultural comparison of disordered eating in Korean women. *International Journal of Eating Disorders,* **39:** 498–502.

*Jennings PS, Forbes D, McDermott B, Hulse G and Juniper S (2006) Eating disorder attitudes and psychopathology in Caucasian Australian, Asian Australian and Thai university students. *Australian and New Zealand Journal of Psychiatry,* **40:** 143–9.

*Jones DC and Crawford JK (2006) The peer appearance culture during adolescence: gender and body mass variations. *Journal of Youth and Adolescence*, **35**: 257–69.

*Kashubeck-West S, Mintz LB and Weigold I. (2005) Separating the effects of gender and weight-loss desire on body satisfaction and disordered eating behavior. *Sex Roles*, **53**: 505–18.

Keel PK and Klump KL (2003) Are eating disorders culture-bound syndromes? Implications for conceptualizing their etiology. *Psychological Bulletin*, **129**: 747–69.

*Keery H, Boutelle K, van den Berg P and Thompson JK (2005) The impact of appearance-related teasing by family members. *Journal of Adolescent Health*, **37**: 120–7.

Klump KL, McGue M and Iacono WG (2000) Age differences in genetic and environmental influences on eating attitudes and behaviors in preadolescent and adolescent female twins. *Journal of Abnormal Psychology*, **109**: 239–51.

*Krones PG, Stice E, Batres C and Orjada K (2005) *In vivo* social comparison to a thin-ideal peer promotes body dissatisfaction: a randomized experiment. *International Journal of Eating Disorders*, **38**: 134–42.

*Kusano-Scharz M and von Wietersheim J (2005) EDI results of Japanese and German women and possible sociocultural explanations. *European Eating Disorders Review*, **13**: 411–16.

*Lamerz A, Kuepper-Nybelen J, Bruning N, Wehle C, Trost-Brinkhues G, Brenner H *et al.* (2005) Prevalence of obesity, binge eating, and night eating in a cross-sectional field survey of 6-year-old children and their parents in a German urban population. *Journal of Child Psychology and Psychiatry*, **46**: 385–93.

*le Grange D, Louw J, Basil R, Nel T and Silkstone C (2006) Eating attitudes and behaviours in South African adolescents and young adults. *Transcultural Psychiatry*, **43**: 401–17.

Levine M, Smolak L and Hayden H (1994) The relation of sociocultural factors to eating attitudes and behaviors among middle school girls. *Journal of Early Adolescence*, **14**: 471–90.

*Lunde C, Frisen A and Hwang CP (2006) Is peer victimization related to body esteem in 10-year-old girls and boys? *Body Image*, **3**: 25–33.

*McCabe MP and Ricciardelli LA (2005a) A longitudinal study of body image and strategies to lose weight and increase muscles among children. *Journal of Applied Developmental Psychology*, **26**: 559–77.

*McCabe MP and Ricciardelli LA (2005b) A prospective study of pressures from parents, peers and the media on extreme weight change behaviors among adolescent boys and girls. *Behavior Research and Therapy*, **43**: 653–68.

*McKinley NM (2006) Longitudinal gender differences in objectified body consciousness and weight-related attitudes and behaviors: cultural and developmental contexts in the transition from college. *Sex Roles*, **54**: 159–73.

*Meyer C, Leung N, Waller G, Perkins S, Paice N and Mitchell J (2005) Anger and bulimic psychopathology: gender differences in a non-clinical group. *International Journal of Eating Disorders*, **37**: 69–71.

*Muris P and Littel M (2005) Domains of childhood teasing and psychopathological symptoms in Dutch adolescents. *Psychological Reports*, **96**: 707–8.

*Muris P, Meesters C, van de Blom W and Mayer B (2005) Biological, psychological and sociocultural correlates of body change strategies and eating problems in adolescent boys and girls. *Eating Behavior*, **6**: 11–22.

*Paxton SJ, Eisenberg ME and Neumark-Sztainer D (2006) Prospective predictors of body dissatisfaction in adolescent girls and boys: a five-year longitudinal study. *Developmental Psychology*, **42**: 888–99.

*Phan T and Tylka TL (2006) Exploring a model and moderators of disordered eating with Asian American college women. *Journal of Counseling Psychology*, **53**: 36–47.

*Reagan P and Hersch J (2005) Influence of race, gender, and socioeconomic status on binge-eating frequency in a population-based sample. *International Journal of Eating Disorders*, **38**: 252–6.

*Regan PC and Cachelin FM (2006) Binge eating and purging in a multi-ethnic community sample. *International Journal of Eating Disorders*, **39**: 523–6.

*Ricciardelli LA, McCabe MP, Lillis J and Thomas K (2006) A longitudinal investigation of the development of weight and muscle concerns among preadolescent boys. *Journal of Youth and Adolescence*, **35**: 177–87.

*Roberts A, Cash TF, Feingold A and Johnson BT (2006) Are black–white differences in females' body dissatisfaction decreasing? A meta-analytic review. *Journal of Consulting and Clinical Psychology*, **74**: 1121–31.

*Rotenberg KJ, Carte L and Speirs A (2005) The effects of modeling dietary restraint on food consumption: do restrained models promote restrained eating? *Eating Behavior*, **6**: 75–84.

*Safir KP, Flaisher-Kellner S and Rosenmann A (2005) When gender differences surpass cultural differences in personal satisfaction with body shape in Israeli college students. *Sex Roles*, **52**: 369–78.

*Sheffield JK, Tse KH and Sofronoff K (2005) A comparison of body-image dissatisfaction and eating disturbance among Australian and Hong Kong women. *European Eating Disorders Review*, **13**: 112–24.

*Shroff H and Thompson JK (2006) Peer influences, body-image dissatisfaction, eating dysfunction and self-esteem in adolescent girls. *Journal of Health Psychology*, **11**: 533–51.

*Smolak L, Murnen SK and Thompson JK (2005) Sociocultural influences and muscle building in adolescent boys. *Psychology of Men and Masculinity*, **6**: 227–39.

*Soh NL, Touyz SW and Surgenor LJ (2006) Eating and body image disturbances across cultures: a review. *European Eating Disorders Review*, **14**: 54–65.

*Stark-Wroblewski K, Yanico BJ and Lupe S (2005) Acculturation, internalization of Western appearance norms, and eating pathology among Japanese and Chinese international student women. *Psychology of Women Quarterly*, **29**: 38–46.

Striegel-Moore RH, Dohm FA, Kraemer HC, Taylor CB, Daniels S, Crawford PB *et al.* (2003) Eating disorders in white and black women. *American Journal of Psychiatry*, **160**: 1326–31.

Striegel-Moore RH, Fairburn CG, Wilfley DE, Pike KM, Dohm FA and Kraemer HC (2005) Toward an understanding of risk factors for binge-eating disorder in black and white women: A community-based case-control study. *Psychological Medicine*, **35**: 907–17.

*Tester ML and Gleaves DH (2005) Self-deceptive enhancement and family environment: possible protective factors against internalization of the thin ideal. *Eating Disorders*, **13**: 187–99.

*van Son GE, van Hoeken D, Bartelds AI, van Furth EF and Hoek HW (2006) Urbanisation and the incidence of eating disorders. *British Journal of Psychiatry*, **189**: 562–3.

*Varnado-Sullivan PJ, Horton R and Savoy S (2006) Differences for gender, weight and exercise in body image disturbance and eating disorder symptoms. *Eating and Weight Disorders*, **11**: 118–25.

***Wardle J, Haase AM and Steptoe A (2006) Body image and weight control in young adults: international comparisons in university students from 22 countries. *International Journal of Obesity*, **30**: 644–51.

This paper included a sample of 18,512 college students from 22 countries, with over 90% participation rates across sites. The results indicate particularly high levels of weight concerns and attempts to lose weight among women in Asian countries.

*Warren CS, Gleaves DH, Cepeda-Benito A, Fernandez Mdel C and Rodriguez-Ruiz S (2005) Ethnicity as a protective factor against internalization of a thin ideal and body dissatisfaction. *International Journal of Eating Disorders*, **37**: 241–9.

*Weltzin TE, Weisensel N, Franczyk D, Burnett K, Klitz C and Bean P (2005) Eating disorders in men: update. *Journal of Men's Health and Gender*, **2**: 186–93.

*Williams LK, Ricciardelli LA, McCabe MP, Waqa GG and Bavadra K (2006) Body image attitudes and concerns among indigenous Fijian and European Australian adolescent girls. *Body Image*, **3**: 275–87.

*York-Crowe EE and Williamson DA (2005) Health and appearance concerns in young Caucasian and African-American women. *Eating and Weight Disorders*, **10**: 38–44.

***Zalta AK and Keel PK (2006) Peer influence on bulimic symptoms in college students. *Journal of Abnormal Psychology*, **115**: 185–9.

This paper utilized a longitudinal, multi-level design to determine how peer selection and socialization influence bulimic symptoms. The results indicate that personal vulnerabilities intersect with the selection of social environments to impact on disordered eating.

4

Epidemiology of eating disorders: an update

Anna Keski-Rahkonen, Anu Raevuori and Hans W Hoek

Abstract

Objectives of review. To summarize the recent advances in the descriptive epidemiology of eating disorders, emphasizing studies published between 2005 and 2006.

Summary of recent findings. During their lifetime, 0.9–2.2% of women and 0.2–0.3% of men suffer from anorexia nervosa (AN). Its overall incidence in the population has remained stable during the 1990s compared with the 1980s, but has increased among adolescent girls. Most recent studies confirm previous findings of high mortality associated with AN. Bulimia nervosa (BN) affects 1.5–2% of women and 0.5% of men, and its occurrence may be decreasing. Atypical eating disorder cases account for the majority of all clinical and community eating disorder cases, and only a minority receive specialized treatment.

Future directions. The incidence and prevalence of AN and BN have been extensively quantified in European and North American settings. However, non-Western populations and atypical manifestations of eating disorders remain a challenge for future studies.

Introduction

Descriptive epidemiological studies provide information about the occurrence of disease and trends in the frequency of disease over time. The most commonly used descriptive measures in epidemiology are incidence, prevalence and mortality.

Incidence relates the number of new cases to the total number of individuals at risk during the specified period. The incidence of eating disorders is usually expressed as the number of new cases per 100 000 person-years of observation time.

Prevalence is the total number of cases as a proportion of the total population at a specific point in time or during a specified period (e.g. one year or a lifetime).

Mortality rates are often used as an indicator of illness severity. The *crude mortality rate* (CMR) is the proportion of deaths within the study population. The *standardized mortality rate* (SMR) is the ratio of deaths observed compared with the expected mortality rate in the population of origin (e.g. all young females).

Mortality rates are by their nature distal outcome measures. More proximal measures of both disease processes and outcomes within the population are often necessary for predicting the course of illness and estimating disease burden. Despite various propositions, definitions of outcome, such as criteria for remission and recovery, remain contentious (Couturier and Lock 2006).

The validity and generalizability of results from epidemiological studies are influenced by the selection of target populations and methods of case detection (Hsu 1996; Hoek and van Hoeken 2003). Because eating disorders are relatively rare among the general population, medical records or case registers of a specific catchment area are often used to obtain a sufficient number of cases. Yet because only a fraction of cases will seek professional help or receive a referral to specialized healthcare services, studies limited to clinical settings may grossly underestimate the occurrence of eating disorders in the community. Differential availability of services and variable methods of case detection may be interpreted as changes in occurrence. Findings based on clinical case registers may also lead to biased conclusions about mortality and other disease outcomes, because clinical samples are often biased towards cases with longer duration and greater severity of illness. Large population-based studies are more representative of the source population and less biased in their conclusions, although they are often extremely expensive and time-consuming to conduct.

Our aim was to summarize recent advances in the descriptive epidemiology of eating disorders, updating previous reviews of the same topic (Hoek and van Hoeken 2003; Hoek 2006). We identified articles through MEDLINE using the search terms 'epidemiology', 'incidence', 'prevalence', 'mortality' or 'outcome' in combination with 'eating disorders', 'anorexia nervosa', 'bulimia nervosa', 'binge eating disorder' or 'EDNOS'. Community or population-based studies published in 2005 and 2006 were emphasized.

Literature review

Anorexia nervosa

Incidence

Incidence rates derived from primary care represent eating disorders at the earliest stage of detection. In the UK, new cases of anorexia nervosa (AN) recorded in the *General Practice Research Database* between 1994 and 2000 (Currin *et al.* 2005) were compared to similar data from 1988–1993 (Turnbull *et al.* 1996).

The age- and sex-adjusted incidence of AN remained remarkably consistent over the two study periods. In 2000, it was 4.7 (95% confidence interval [CI]: 3.6–5.8) per 100 000 person-years, compared with 4.2 (95% CI: 3.4–5.0) per 100 000 person-years in 1993.

The incidence of AN ascertained by general practitioners in a large representative sample of the Dutch population was 7.7 (95% CI: 5.9–10.0) per 100 000 person-years during 1995–1999 (van Son *et al.* 2006a), practically the same as the rate of 7.4 per 100 000 person-years during 1985–1989. Incidence rates for AN were considerably higher for females aged 15–19 years, accounting for 40% of all identified cases resulting in an incidence of 109 per 100 000 in this age group (Hoek and van Hoeken 2003).

In Switzerland, the incidence rate of cases admitted for AN was 20 per 100 000 person-years for females between 12 and 25 years of age during 1993–1995 (Milos *et al.* 2004).

The sole recent effort known to us to quantify rates of AN directly in the general population yielded an incidence of 270 per 100 000 person-years among 15–19 year old Finnish female twins during the period 1990–1998 (Keski-Rahkonen *et al.* 2007). This community rate is much higher than the rate of 109 per 100 000 15–19 year old females in general practice in the Netherlands during 1995–1999 (van Son *et al.* 2006a), probably because the Finnish study was conducted in the community rather than through primary health care. If we combine the Finnish incidence rate in the community with the Dutch rate in general practice, only 43% (109/270) of all community cases have been detected. This percentage is similar to the finding of 40% reported in a meta-analysis by Hoek (2006).

Prevalence

The lifetime prevalence of AN diagnosed according to the *Diagnostic and Statistical Manual of Mental Disorders, Fourth Edition (DSM-IV)* was 1.2% among women in the 1935–1958 birth cohorts of Swedish twins (Bulik *et al.* 2006). The lifetime prevalence of broad DSM-IV AN, defined as DSM-IV AN excluding amenorrhea, in the same study was an additional 1.2%. In an Australian study of female twins aged 28–39 years, the lifetime prevalence of AN was 1.9%, with an additional 2.4% for partial AN (i.e. anorexia in the absence of amenorrhea) (Wade *et al.* 2006). The lifetime prevalence of DSM-IV AN was 2.2% in a large sample of women from the 1975–1979 birth cohorts of Finnish twins (Keski-Rahkonen *et al.* 2007), and an additional 2% of women fulfilled the criteria for ICD-10 atypical anorexia. In a nationally representative survey of the US household population, the lifetime prevalence of DSM-IV AN was found to be 0.9% among adult females (Hudson *et al.* 2007). Thus, according to various methodologically sound, large-scale, nationally representative surveys, 0.9–2.2% of women in Western countries suffer from DSM-IV AN during their lifetime. Forms of AN that fall below the diagnostic threshold appear to be about twice as common.

In a recent nationwide study conducted in Portugal among adolescent girls aged 12–23 years, the point prevalence of DSM-IV AN was 0.39% (Machado *et al.* 2006). An Austrian community-based questionnaire survey (Mangweth-Matzek *et al.* 2006) assessed AN among women aged 50–60 years. AN was rare among the elderly – only one participant met the DSM-IV criteria for AN, yielding a point prevalence of 0.2%.

Time trends

The registered incidence of AN increased in Europe until the 1970s, but seems to have remained relatively stable thereafter (Hoek 2006). The study of Swedish twins born during the period 1935–1958 (Bulik *et al.* 2006) documented a clear increase in the prevalence of DSM-IV AN in both sexes among participants born after 1945. In the Netherlands, the overall incidence of AN has been otherwise stable, but increased significantly (from 56.4 to 109.2 per 100 000) among 15–19 year old females from 1985–1989 to 1995–1999 (van Son *et al.* 2006a). In Switzerland, the changes in incidence of first-time hospitalization of females with AN were studied in a geographically defined region using the same medical-record-based methodology from 1956 to 1995. The incidence of severe AN increased significantly during the 1960s and 1970s, but appears to have reached a plateau of around 1.2 per 100 000 person-years thereafter (Milos *et al.* 2004).

Mortality

In the 1990s, AN was associated with the highest rate of mortality of all mental disorders (Harris and Barraclough 1998). Recent studies have confirmed the high mortality rate within the AN patient population. In Canada, 326 patients diagnosed with AN completed an assessment over a 20-year period, and the SMR was 10.5 (95% CI: 5.5–15.5) (Birmingham *et al.* 2005). In northeast Scotland, 23 out of 524 patients with AN who were seen in specialist services died, and the median length of time between diagnosis and death was 11 years (Millar *et al.* 2005). The CMR in this study was 4.4% and the SMR was 3.3 (95% CI: 2.2–4.9). AN was only mentioned on the death certificate in one-third of the cases, but eating disorders or other psychiatric pathology probably contributed to several of the other deaths. In a 12-year follow-up study of 103 patients with AN in Germany, the CMR was 7.7%, and a further 40% of patients had a poor outcome (Fichter *et al.* 2006).

In a recent Swedish study (Lindblad *et al.* 2006), a significantly higher mortality rate (4.4% vs. 1.2%) was found among female patients hospitalized due to AN in 1977–1981 compared with those hospitalized in 1987–1991. The hazard ratio of death for the 1977–1981 cohort relative to the 1987–1991 cohort was 3.7. Lindblad *et al.* (2006) argue that this dramatic decrease in the mortality rate is related to the introduction of specialized care units for patients with eating disorders.

However, a Norwegian study based on national patient and cause of death registers found rates of AN-related deaths to be 6.5 and 9.9 per 100 000 (Reas *et al.* 2005). Of the documented deaths, 44% occurred at or above the age of 65 years, implying that many AN patients have a relatively long life expectancy. An earlier population-based study (Korndorfer *et al.* 2003) of all patients presenting with AN in Rochester, Minnesota, in 1935–1989 found an estimated survival rate of 93% 30 years after the initial diagnosis of AN, which did not differ significantly from an expected population survival rate of 94%. The SMR was 0.71 (95% CI: 0.42–1.09).

Finally, in an audit conducted in the UK, death certificates emerged as a flawed source of information. Both over-reporting and under-reporting of AN as a cause of death occurred, the latter probably being more common (Muir and Palmer 2004).

Other illness outcomes

Several new community or population cohort-based epidemiological studies have focused on outcomes other than mortality in AN. Long-term recovery rates from AN were relatively good – the five-year recovery rate from DSM-IV AN was 66% (Keski-Rahkonen *et al.* 2007). Residual symptoms were very frequent (Wade *et al.* 2006; Keski-Rahkonen *et al.* 2007), but appeared to progress to full recovery over time (Keski-Rahkonen *et al.* 2007). Although AN is often perceived as a chronic illness, its mean duration among the general population is shorter than was previously thought, at 1.7 years in the USA (Hudson *et al.* 2007) and three years in Finland (Keski-Rahkonen *et al.* 2007). Only a minority of cases of AN seek treatment (Hoek 2006; Hudson *et al.* 2007; Keski-Rahkonen *et al.* 2007).

Males

Although AN occurs in males as well as in females, only a few studies have reported its incidence among males. In the Netherlands and the UK, the incidence of AN among males was less than 1 per 100 000 person-years (Currin *et al.* 2005; van Son *et al.* 2006a). However, according to recent Swedish, Finnish and American population studies, AN in males appears to be more common. In a large-scale, population-based study of Swedish twin birth cohorts for the period 1945–1958 (Bulik *et al.* 2006), the prevalence of DSM-IV AN in males was 0.11%. No cases of male AN were detected in the birth cohorts for the period 1935–1944. Combining clinical interview data with Swedish Hospital Discharge Register and National Cause of Death Register data, the lifetime prevalence of AN in males was found to be 0.29%.

In Finland, a lifetime prevalence of 0.24% for DSM-IV AN was detected among young men aged 22–27 years (Raevuori *et al.* 2007). The incidence of DSM-IV AN among 12–25 year old males was 18 per 100 000 person-years.

In a nationally representative survey of US households (Hudson *et al.* 2007), the lifetime prevalence of DSM-IV AN was found to be 0.3% among men. Based on figures in these studies, the rough rate ratio of females compared with males is between four and 10. Thus, many recent community-based studies have found that AN is more common among males than previously thought. AN may be even more frequently underdetected in males than in females.

Non-Western countries

Abnormal eating attitudes and behaviors are frequent in developing countries and among ethnic minorities, particularly among individuals of Asian and African descent (Becker *et al.* 2005; Pike and Mizushima 2005; Striegel-Moore *et al.* 2005; Tong *et al.* 2005). Recent studies demonstrate that AN does occur in non-Western countries (Lee *et al.* 2005; Uzun *et al.* 2006). The most comprehensive attempt to quantify eating disorders in non-Western settings took place on the Caribbean island of Curaçao, where the full spectrum of community health service providers was contacted (Hoek *et al.* 2005). The overall incidence of AN was 1.82 (95% CI: 0.74–2.89) per 100 000 person-years, much lower than that in the USA and Western Europe. No cases were found among the majority black population. However, among the minority mixed and white population the incidence resembled that in the Netherlands and the USA.

Bulimia nervosa

Incidence and time trends

In the Netherlands, the nationwide primary care-based study (van Son *et al.* 2006a) found a statistically non-significant decreasing trend in the incidence of BN when comparing two five-year periods, namely 1985–1989 (incidence rate 8.6 per 100 000 person-years) and 1995–1999 (incidence rate 6.1 per 100 000 person-years). Compared with rural areas, the incidence of BN was almost 2.5 times higher in urbanized areas and five times higher in large cities (van Son *et al.* 2006b).

In the UK, the age-adjusted and sex-adjusted incidence of BN in primary care decreased during the second half of the 1990s from 12.2 per 100 000 person-years in 1993 to 6.6 per 100 000 person-years in 2000 (95% CI: 5.3–7.9) (Currin *et al.* 2005). This possible decrease in the occurrence of BN is also supported by some recent evidence provided by an American study of college students, which suggests that the point prevalence of BN among women has significantly decreased over two decades, from 4.2% in 1982 to 1.3% in 1992 and 1.7% in 2002 (Keel *et al.* 2006). Based on recent studies, it thus appears that the peak of the bulimia epidemic was reached by the early 1990s, and that rates of bulimia have started to decrease since then.

Prevalence

The generally accepted prevalence rate of BN from two-stage studies is about 1% among young females (Hoek and van Hoeken 2003). The lifetime prevalence was 2.0% for BN according to DSM-IV criteria in a large sample of women from the 1975–1979 birth cohorts of Finnish twins (Keski-Rahkonen *et al.* 2006), and the point prevalence for DSM-IV BN in the sample was 0.9%. A representative survey of the US household population (Hudson *et al.* 2007) found that the lifetime prevalence of DSM-IV BN was 1.5% in adult females. In adolescent female populations, the prevalence of BN is often still lower than among adult women. In a nationwide study in Portugal, the prevalence of DSM-IV BN among 12–23 year old females (mean age 16 years) was only 0.3% (Machado *et al.* 2006). In a Spanish study (Rodriguez-Cano *et al.* 2005) of 13–15 year old adolescents representing the general population, the prevalence of BN according to ICD-10, DSM-III-R and DSM-IV criteria was 0.75% among girls. Thus, bulimia affects 1–2% of young women during their lifetime. However, as bulimic symptoms often have a later onset than anorexic symptoms, the prevalence of bulimia is generally lower among adolescent women than among young adult women.

Mortality

Few studies have assessed mortality associated with BN. A meta-analysis encompassing 43 follow-up studies of BN cohorts gave an overall aggregate SMR of 1.6 (95% CI: 0.8–2.7) for BN (Nielsen 2003).

Males

The lifetime prevalence of DSM-IV BN was found to be 0.5% among adult males in the USA (Hudson *et al.* 2007), somewhat higher than expected on the basis of earlier reports (Hoek and van Hoeken 2003).

Eating disorders not otherwise specified (EDNOS)

Currently, in outpatient settings, 15% of cases present with AN and 25% present with BN. EDNOS accounts for the remaining 60% of cases (Fairburn and Bohn 2005). The category EDNOS includes partial syndromes of AN and BN. Despite demonstrating a core cognitive psychopathology similar to other eating disorder sufferers, EDNOS patients represent the least studied group of patients with eating disorders. The prevalence of EDNOS according to DSM-IV criteria was 2.4% in a nationwide study of Portuguese female students aged 12–23 years. EDNOS accounted for 77% of all diagnosed cases of eating disorders in the community (Machado *et al.* 2006). In a Spanish study of 13–15 year old adolescents from the general population, the prevalence of EDNOS was 4.9% in females and 0.6% in males (Rodriguez-Cano *et al.* 2005). An Austrian questionnaire survey (Mangweth-Matzek *et al.* 2006) examined a randomly selected non-clinical sample of elderly women. In total, 3.8% of the women met the criteria for eating disorders, and the great majority of them (15/18) were diagnosed with EDNOS.

Binge-eating disorder (BED)

In a nationally representative study conducted in the USA, the lifetime prevalence of DSM-IV BED was 3.5% among adult females and 2.0% among adult males (Hudson *et al.* 2007). BED occurs frequently among black women, but may be even more common among white women (Striegel-Moore *et al.* 2005). Although BED has traditionally been associated with obesity, it appears to aggregate strongly in families independently of obesity (Hudson *et al.* 2006).

Clinical implications and summary of important findings

AN is generally considered to be a rare disorder, but recent community studies suggest that its lifetime prevalence may be higher than previously thought (up to 2% among women and 0.3% among men). Some recent evidence suggests that the incidence of BN is decreasing, but atypical forms of eating disorders, such as BED and EDNOS, appear to be very common in the community. Most individuals with eating disorders do not seek specialized care. Thus, there is an ongoing need to train community healthcare providers to improve their detection of eating disorders.

Recent studies show that the mortality rate of AN is still very high, and probably the highest of all the mental disorders. The availability of specialized care for patients with eating disorders may decrease mortality from AN. Yet studies that focus on individuals receiving clinical care may bias conclusions about the prognosis of eating disorders. Recent population-based studies of AN have revealed that recovery rates are relatively favorable, and that the mean duration of illness may be shorter than was previously thought.

Future directions

Recent large population-based studies of North Americans and Europeans have extensively quantified the incidence and prevalence of AN and BN using reliable standardized methods. Yet the incidence and prevalence of eating disorders appear to be changing rapidly among non-Western populations, where their documentation remains a challenge.

Although mortality associated with AN has received much attention, the natural course of eating disorders remains poorly understood. More proximal outcomes should be systematically assessed and reported.

The large majority of all eating disorder cases in both outpatient settings and the community fall into the heterogeneous category EDNOS. As current diagnostic classifications have failed to capture adequately the commonest forms of eating disorders, current diagnostic boundaries may require radical rethinking and refining in the future.

The scope of this review has been limited to descriptive epidemiology. However, the future of epidemiological research lies in analytical epidemiology – that is, understanding more fully the risk factors and etiological mechanisms of eating disorders. Promising areas of inquiry include genetic, epigenetic and cultural mechanisms in the development of eating disorders.

References

(References included from the targeted review years are preceded by one asterisk. References preceded by three asterisks are of particular significance. The significance is explained by a short commentary following the complete reference.)

*Becker AE, Gilman SE and Burwell RA (2005) Changes in prevalence of overweight and in body image among Fijian women between 1989 and 1998. *Obesity Research*, **13**: 110–17.

*Birmingham CL, Su J, Hlynsky JA, Goldner EM and Gao M (2005) The mortality rate from anorexia nervosa. *International Journal of Eating Disorders*, **38**: 143–6.

***Bulik CM, Sullivan PF, Tozzi F, Furberg H, Lichtenstein P and Pedersen NL (2006) Prevalence, heritability, and prospective risk factors for anorexia nervosa. *Archives of General Psychiatry*, **63**: 305–12.

This is the largest twin study ever conducted in individuals with rigorously diagnosed AN in a population-based sample of Swedish twins born between 1935 and 1958. The prevalence of AN was higher in individuals of both sexes born after 1945. Prospectively assessed neuroticism was associated with the subsequent development of AN.

*Couturier J and Lock J (2006) What is recovery in adolescent anorexia nervosa? *International Journal of Eating Disorders*, **39**: 550–55.

***Currin L, Schmidt U, Treasure J and Jick H (2005) Time trends in eating disorder incidence. *British Journal of Psychiatry*, **186**: 132–5.

This study examined time trends in eating disorders at primary care level in the UK during the years 1994–2000. The incidence of AN remained constant over the period studied. There was an increase in the incidence of BN, but rates declined after a peak in 1996.

***Fairburn CG and Bohn K (2005) Eating disorder NOS (EDNOS): an example of the troublesome "not otherwise specified" (NOS) category in DSM-IV. *Behavior Research and Therapy*, **43**: 691–701.

This analysis of four well-diagnosed adult samples of patients with eating disorders showed that EDNOS is the commonest eating disorder in outpatient settings.

*Fichter MM, Quadflieg N and Hedlund S (2006) Twelve-year course and outcome predictors of anorexia nervosa. *International Journal of Eating Disorders*, **39**: 87–100.

Harris EC and Barraclough B (1998) Excess mortality of mental disorder. *British Journal of Psychiatry*, **173**: 11–53.

*Hoek HW (2006) Incidence, prevalence and mortality of anorexia nervosa and other eating disorders. *Current Opinions in Psychiatry*, **19**: 389–94.

Hoek HW and van Hoeken D (2003) Review of the prevalence and incidence of eating disorders. *International Journal of Eating Disorders*, **34**: 383–96.

***Hoek HW, van Harten PN, Hermans KME, Katzman MA, Matroos GE and Susser ES (2005) The incidence of anorexia nervosa on Curaçao. *American Journal of Psychiatry*, **162**: 748–52.

This comprehensive epidemiological study was conducted on a Caribbean island with a mainly black population. It was found that on Curaçao, sociocultural factors appear to be associated with differential incidence rates of AN.

Hsu LKG (1996) Epidemiology of the eating disorders. *Psychiatric Clinics of North America*, **19**: 681–700.

*Hudson JI, Lalonde JK, Berry JM, Pindyck LJ, Bulik CM, Crow SJ *et al.* (2006) Binge-eating disorder as a distinct familial phenotype in obese individuals. *Archives of General Psychiatry*, **63**: 313–19.

***Hudson JI, Hiripi E, Pope HG Jr. and Kessler RC (2007) The prevalence and correlates of eating disorders in the national comorbidity survey replication. *Biological Psychiatry*, **61**: 348–58.

This large nationally representative study from the USA documents the 12-month prevalence of eating disorders and also attempts to quantify comorbidity and impairment associated with eating disorders.

*Keel PK, Heatherton TF, Dorer DJ, Joiner TE and Zalta AK (2006) Point prevalence of bulimia nervosa in 1982, 1992 and 2002. *Psychological Medicine*, **36**: 119–27.

*Keski-Rahkonen A, Sihvola E, Raevuori A, Kaukoranta J, Bulik CM, Hoek HW *et al.* (2006) Reliability of self-reported eating disorders: optimizing population screening. *International Journal of Eating Disorders*, **39**: 754–62.

***Keski-Rahkonen A, Hoek HW, Susser ES, Linna MS, Sihvola E, Raevuori A *et al.* (2007) Epidemiology and course of anorexia nervosa in the community. *American Journal of Psychiatry*, **164**: 1259–65.

This nationwide Finnish twin study of young adult women found a substantially higher lifetime prevalence and incidence of DSM-IV AN than has previously been reported. The 5-year clinical recovery rates were better than those in most previous studies.

Korndorfer SR, Lucas AR, Suman VJ, Crowson CS, Krahn LE and Melton LJ (2003) Long-term survival of patients with anorexia nervosa: a population-based study in Rochester, Minn. *Mayo Clinic Proceedings*, **78**: 278–84.

*Lee HY, Lee EL, Pathy P and Chan YH (2005) Anorexia nervosa in Singapore: an eight-year retrospective study. *Singapore Medical Journal*, **46**: 275–81.

*Lindblad F, Lindberg L and Hjern A (2006) Improved survival in adolescent patients with anorexia nervosa: a comparison of two Swedish national cohorts of female inpatients. *American Journal of Psychiatry*, **163**: 1433–5.

*Machado PP, Machado BC, Goncalves S and Hoek HW (2006) The prevalence of eating disorders not otherwise specified. *International Journal of Eating Disorders*, **40**: 212–17.

*Mangweth-Matzek B, Rupp CI, Hausmann A, Assmayr K, Mariacher E, Kemmler G *et al.* (2006) Never too old for eating disorders or body dissatisfaction: a community study of elderly women. *International Journal of Eating Disorders*, **39**: 583–6.

*Millar HR, Wardell F, Vyvyan JP, Naji SA, Prescott GJ and Eagles JM (2005) Anorexia nervosa mortality in Northeast Scotland, 1965–1999. *American Journal of Psychiatry*, **162**: 753–7.

Milos G, Spindler A, Schnyder U, Martz J, Hoek HW and Willi J (2004) Incidence of severe anorexia nervosa in Switzerland: 40 years of development. *International Journal of Eating Disorders*, **35**: 250–58.

Muir A and Palmer RL (2004) An audit of a British sample of death certificates in which anorexia nervosa is listed as a cause of death. *International Journal of Eating Disorders*, **36**: 356–60.

Nielsen S (2003) Standardized mortality ratio in bulimia nervosa. *Archives of General Psychiatry*, **60**: 851.

*Pike KM and Mizushima H (2005) The clinical presentation of Japanese women with anorexia nervosa and bulimia nervosa: a study of the Eating Disorders Inventory-2. *International Journal of Eating Disorders*, **37**: 26–31.

Raevuori A, Hoek HW, Rissanen A, Kaprio J and Keski-Rahkonen A (2007) *Incidence and lifetime prevalence of anorexia nervosa in young men.* Paper presented at the International Conference on Eating Disorders, Baltimore, Maryland, 2–5 May 2007.

*Reas DL, Kjelsas E, Heggestad T, Eriksen L, Nielsen S, Gjertsen F *et al.* (2005) Character-istics of anorexia nervosa-related deaths in Norway (1992–2000): data from the National Patient Register and the Causes of Death Register. *International Journal of Eating Disorders*, **37**: 181–7.

*Rodriguez-Cano T, Beato-Fernandez L and Belmonte-Llario A (2005) New contributions to the prevalence of eating disorders in Spanish adolescents: detection of false negatives. *European Psychiatry*, **20**: 173–8.

*Striegel-Moore RH, Fairburn CG, Wilfley DE, Pike KM, Dohm FA and Kraemer HC (2005) Toward an understanding of risk factors for binge-eating disorder in black and white women: a community-based case–control study. *Psychological Medicine*, **35**: 907–17.

*Tong J, Miao SJ, Wang J, Zhang JJ, Wu HM, Li T *et al.* (2005) Five cases of male eating disorders in Central China. *International Journal of Eating Disorders*, **37**: 72–5.

Turnbull S, Ward A, Treasure J, Jick H and Derby L (1996) The demand for eating disorder care. An epidemiological study using the General Practice Research Database. *British Journal of Psychiatry*, **169**: 705–12.

*Uzun O, Gulec N, Ozsahin A, Doruk A, Ozdemir B and Caliskan U (2006) Screening disordered eating attitudes and eating disorders in a sample of Turkish female college students. *Comprehensive Psychiatry*, **47**: 123–6.

***van Son GE, van Hoeken D, Bartelds AI, van Furth EF and Hoek HW (2006a) Time trends in the incidence of eating disorders: a primary care study in the Netherlands. *International Journal of Eating Disorders*, **39**: 565–9.

This Dutch primary care-based study examined changes in the incidence of eating disorders in the 1990s compared to the 1980s. The increase of incidence of anorexia nervosa among the high risk group continued to the end of the past century, but the incidence of bulimia did not rise as expected.

*van Son GE, van Hoeken D, Bartelds AI, van Furth EF and Hoek HW (2006b) Urbanisation and the incidence of eating disorders. *British Journal of Psychiatry*, **189**: 562–3.

*Wade TD, Bergin JL, Tiggemann M, Bulik CM and Fairburn CG (2006) Prevalence and long-term course of lifetime eating disorders in an adult Australian twin cohort. *Australian and New Zealand Journal of Psychiatry*, **40**: 121–8.

5

Body image

Susan J Paxton and Brooke E Heinicke

Abstract

Objectives of review. The objective of this review was to summarize major research contributions in the body image field published in 2005 and 2006, and to consider their clinical implications.

Summary of recent findings. The early emergence of body dissatisfaction in children has been documented, and new assessment instruments have enhanced our capacity to assess the multifaceted nature of body image. Prospective research has identified social, psychological and genetic risk factors for body dissatisfaction. However, body dissatisfaction increases risk for negative affect as well as disordered eating. Selective prevention programs have shown mixed results, whilst the efficacy of targeted interventions has been strongly supported. Recent research provides strong support for cognitive–behavioral interventions for body dissatisfaction, and the use of modern technologies shows great promise for extending access to interventions.

Future directions. Although the groundwork has been laid, the greatest research challenge remains the development and evaluation of effective prevention interventions.

Introduction

With the aid of electronic databases we identified over 600 empirical articles, published in peer-reviewed journals during 2005 and 2006, that addressed aspects of body image. We have attempted to distill from this literature the major themes of the issues addressed and directions and developments in the field. We have reviewed significant research contributions under the following categories: prevalence and developmental trends; assessment of body image; psychosocial correlates and risk factors for body image; male body image; negative impact of poor body image; and intervention for body dissatisfaction. We conclude our review by exploring future directions in this area of research.

Literature review

Prevalence and developmental trends

A notable recent development in the body image literature has been the growing interest in body image in children. Dohnt and Tiggemann (2006a) examined body image attitudes in girls from reception (the year preceding grade 1) to grade 3. In reception, 48.4% of girls wished to have a larger body. However, in grade 1, 46.7% wished to be thinner, and this level remained quite constant over the following two years. Despite the desire to be thinner, 45.0% and 48.0% of girls described themselves as 'always' or 'usually' happy, respectively, with their appearance. Thus, cognitive and affective aspects of body image appear to be distinct in this age group. In boys aged 8–11 years, 47.4% wished to be thinner whereas 20.7% wished to have a larger body (Ricciardelli et al. 2006). Rasnake et al. (2005) studied 11–14 year old girls and boys and observed that 57.0% of girls, compared with 32.7% of boys, wished to be thinner, whereas 34.6% of boys, compared with 10.9% of girls, wished to have a larger body. Clearly, the foundation for body dissatisfaction is being laid very early in life.

Prospective research into change in body image during adolescence supports an upward trend in dissatisfaction in girls until late adolescence. Over a two-year period in adolescent girls, Bearman et al. (2006) observed an increase in body dissatisfaction (i.e. scores corresponding to 'moderately dissatisfied' or 'extremely dissatisfied') from 37% to 44%. However, in boys they observed a decrease in dissatisfaction from 23% to 16%. Eisenberg et al. (2006) examined change in body satisfaction among adolescents (mean age at baseline 14.9 years) over a five-year period. Body satisfaction decreased from early to middle adolescence in girls and boys, and also from middle adolescence to young adulthood in boys but not in girls. In younger adolescents, among certain ethnic groups of males and among those whose body mass index (BMI) increased during the five-year period, larger decreases in satisfaction were observed.

Within the USA, research with adolescents and young women has continued into differences in body image between ethnic subcultures in community-based samples (e.g. Kelly et al. 2005) and eating disorder samples (e.g. White and Grilo 2005). Grabe and Hyde (2006) reviewed a large literature in a meta-analysis and concluded that white women, especially during adolescence and young adulthood, had significantly higher levels of body dissatisfaction than black women, but this difference was small ($d = 0.29$), and Hispanic women had higher levels of dissatisfaction than black women ($d = 0.18$). However, there was no difference in dissatisfaction levels between white and Asian American women or between white and Hispanic women. The authors challenge the notion that body dissatisfaction is predominantly a white woman's problem.

Body image research has been extended into developing and non-Western cultures. Notably, levels of body dissatisfaction in these cultures are typically comparable to those in Western cultures. One example of this research is a study by McArthur et al. (2005) of 12–19 year old girls and boys in six Latin American cities. They found that 49% of girls and 33% of boys wished to be thinner. In a study of Chinese children and adolescents aged 3–15 years ($n = 9100$), Li et al.

(2005) concluded that levels of body dissatisfaction were not dissimilar to those found in developed countries. Overweight girls and boys tended to be dissatisfied with their bodies at nine and 11 years of age, respectively. In both sexes, body satisfaction, mild dissatisfaction and moderate dissatisfaction rates were 40.1%, 36.4% and 23.5%, respectively. Body image research has also been conducted in countries as diverse as Gambia (e.g. Siervo *et al.* 2006), Korea (e.g. Jung and Lee 2006) and Oman (e.g. Al-Adawi *et al.* 2006).

Although much attention has recently been focused on body image issues in children and adolescents, some researchers are now examining the role of body image in older populations. A recent study of body image concerns in women aged between 60 and 70 years found that over 60% of them were dissatisfied with their bodies, and more than 80% of the women controlled their weight (Mangweth-Matzek *et al.* 2006).

Finally, the issue of whether body dissatisfaction has increased over time in different communities has been investigated. A study of two cohorts of Norwegian adolescents, in which data from the first cohort was collected in 1992 and data from the second cohort was collected 10 years later in 2002, found an increase in the proportion of adolescents who were dissatisfied, as well in the proportion who were very satisfied, with their appearance during this period (Storvoll *et al.* 2005). The authors concluded that the increased proportion of adolescents with a negative body image could partly be explained by an increase in BMI over the same period. In a dramatically different environment, in girls in Fiji, body dissatisfaction increased over a 10-year period independent of BMI (Becker *et al.* 2005). This change may reflect a shift in prevailing cultural beliefs associated with modernization.

Assessment

In recognition of the multi-dimensional nature of body image and the need to explore these dimensions further using instruments with demonstrated reliability and validity, there has been a rapid increase in the number of assessment instruments that have been developed over the last two years.

Body-image-related experiences, beliefs and attitudes

Previous research has demonstrated the negative impact of weight-related teasing on body image. The development and validation of the Verbal Commentary on Physical Appearance Scale (Herbozo and Thompson 2006) will facilitate the assessment of both positive and negative verbal commentary about appearance, including negative comments on weight and shape, positive comments on weight and shape, and positive comments on general appearance.

The increasing focus of attention on the complexity of body image is illustrated by scales that have been developed and validated to assess both positive aspects of body image, such as body appreciation (Body Appreciation Scale; Avalos *et al.* 2005), and negative aspects, such as uneasiness felt about one's body (Body Uneasiness Test; Cuzzolaro *et al.* 2006). Appreciation of this complexity has extended to recognition of the need for culturally appropriate scales. For example, the Negative Physical Self Scale was designed to assess body dissatisfaction in the Chinese population, which frequently concerns general appearance, facial appearance and short stature, rather than being overweight (Chen *et al.* 2006). Potentially useful in both therapeutic and research settings, the Body Image Cognitive Distortions scale has been designed to assess eight types of distorted thinking related to how people process information about their physical appearance (Jakatdar *et al.* 2006).

Research focused on body image concerns in males has highlighted the need to develop appropriate instruments for male samples. In response to this, measures of men's attitudes towards their bodies, with a focus on muscularity, low body fat and height (Male Body Attitudes Scale; Tylka *et al.* 2005), attitudes towards muscularity (Swansea Muscularity Attitudes Questionnaire; Wojtowicz and von Ranson 2006), and social and cultural influences on male body image (Questionnaire on Influences on Male Body Shape Model; Toro *et al.* 2005), have been developed.

Body-image-related behaviors

Body dissatisfaction is not only manifested in terms of beliefs and attitudes, but also underpins behaviors. Cash *et al.* (2005) examined the reliability and validity of the Body Image Coping Strategies Inventory (BICSI), an inventory designed to assess how individuals typically manage challenges or threats to body image experiences. The measure was valid, internally consistent, and converged well with other key body image variables and psychosocial functioning measures.

Adding to the limited assessment measures for dysmorphic concerns, Littleton *et al.* (2005a) developed and validated a brief self-report measure designed to assess dysmorphic concern, known as the Body Image Concern Inventory (BICI). This includes items related to body dissatisfaction, checking and camouflaging behavior, and interference due to symptoms. The Body Influence Assessment Inventory (BIAI) (Osman *et al.* 2006), a measure that assesses four dimensions of bodily experiences related to eating disorders that are linked with suicide-related behaviors, has also been developed and undergone initial validation, and shows good preliminary psychometric properties.

Psychosocial correlates and risk factors for body image

Children

There have been important developments regarding identification of correlates and risk factors for body dissatisfaction in children. Cross-sectional research confirms that in pre-adolescent children, body dissatisfaction is positively associated with BMI (e.g. for girls, see Clark and Tiggemann 2006; for boys, see Ricciardelli *et al.* 2006). A path analysis conducted in a cross-sectional sample of 9–12 year old girls supports the crucial role of sociocultural influences on body image, even at this age (Clark and Tiggemann 2006). Clark and Tiggemann observed a significant path from peer appearance conversations to internalization of the thin ideal, which was in turn significantly related to body dissatisfaction. Lunde *et al.* (2006) identified a positive association between body dissatisfaction and non-appearance-related peer victimization in 10-year-old girls and boys.

Experimental and prospective designs provide support for possible causal links between sociocultural variables and body dissatisfaction in children. One experimental study observed the impact on the body image of 5.5–8.5 year old girls of exposure to images of a Barbie doll, an Emme doll (a US size 16) or neutral pictures, each presented to illustrate the same story (Dittmar *et al.* 2006). The 5.5–6.5 year old and 6.5–7.5 year old age groups, but not the 7.5–8.5 year old age group, had significantly lower body satisfaction following exposure to a Barbie doll than following exposure to an Emme doll. This research suggests that body satisfaction is affected by exposure to cultural ideals at a very young age. It also suggests that there are ages at which girls are particularly susceptible to Barbie as an aspirational role model (Dittmar *et al.* 2006). A one-year prospective study of 5–8 year old girls was especially innovative in shedding light on risk factors for body dissatisfaction at this young age (Dohnt and Tiggemann 2006b). This research identified the sociocultural variables of perceived peer desire for thinness and appearance television exposure (i.e. exposure to television which has an emphasis on appearance and the thin ideal) as prospective predictors of appearance satisfaction after controlling for baseline body dissatisfaction.

Adolescents

Examination of correlates of body dissatisfaction during adolescence has further demonstrated positive relationships between poor body image and personal attributes such as negative affect (e.g. Sim and Zeman 2006), endorsement of social attitudes such as internalization of the thin ideal (e.g. Cafri *et al.* 2005), and perceived social pressures such as pressure to be thin (Cafri *et al.* 2005) in girls, and parental appearance messages (Stanford and McCabe 2005), perceived media influence and endorsement of male physical attributes (Smolak and Stein 2006) in boys.

However, during this period the processes involved in the development of body dissatisfaction have also been explored, using cross-sectional, prospective and experimental methodologies. In a cross-sectional study of adolescent girls, Shroff and Thompson (2006) found support for a model in which the effect of peer and media influences on body dissatisfaction was mediated by body comparison and internalization of the thin ideal. Also in girls, Paxton *et al.* (2005) examined the relationships between body dissatisfaction and concerns about boys, and observed direct paths from low self-esteem and depression to body dissatisfaction, but also indirect paths, such that there was a path from low self-esteem to depression, from depression to a strong belief in the importance of popularity with boys, to a belief that thinness is important in attractiveness to boys, and finally to body dissatisfaction. Taken together, these studies suggest that low self-esteem and negative affect may make girls vulnerable to pressures from peers and the media about appearance, which may lead to internalization of beliefs about the importance of thinness to attractiveness, and a greater likelihood of making body comparisons, with the outcome of body dissatisfaction.

Recent research provides greater clarity with regard to prospective risk factors for body dissatisfaction. A two-year prospective study of adolescent girls and boys indicated that initially high levels of negative affect, dietary restraint and deficits in parental support, but not internalization of the thin ideal or BMI, predicted increases in body dissatisfaction (Bearman *et al.* 2006). In a study over a similar time period in Native American adolescents, baseline BMI, anxiety/depression, low self-esteem, lower perceived peer acceptance and lower ethnic identity in boys prospectively predicted body dissatisfaction (Newman *et al.* 2006). In a five-year follow-up study controlling for baseline body dissatisfaction, Paxton *et al.* (2006a) found that baseline BMI, friend dieting and low self-esteem in early adolescent girls, BMI, socioeconomic status (SES) and weight teasing in early adolescent boys, BMI, SES and low self-esteem in middle adolescent girls, and BMI, ethnicity and depression in middle adolescent boys were prospective risk factors for body dissatisfaction five years later. In contrast to observations in younger children, in a one-year prospective study of middle adolescent girls, Tiggemann (2005a) found that media exposure did not predict increased body dissatisfaction at one-year follow-up.

Young adults

In recent years, a large body of research has extended our understanding of factors associated with the development of body dissatisfaction in adult women. Correlates of adult body dissatisfaction (without controlling for baseline body dissatisfaction) and, of particular interest, the genetic contribution to body dissatisfaction were examined using twin modeling (Keski-Rahkonen *et al.* 2005). Correlates of adult body dissatisfaction were early onset of puberty, early initiation of sexual activity, and multiple sexual partners. In women, body dissatisfaction showed moderate to high heritability, whereas in men it was purely environmental. However, this study could not assess the potential genetic overlap between BMI and body dissatisfaction.

A strong focus of research into body dissatisfaction has been the role of peer and media influences. In experimental studies, Britton *et al.* (2006) demonstrated that, in women, self-denigrating 'fat talk' amongst friends was normative behavior, while Krones *et al.* (2005) showed that women who were exposed to a thin compared with an average-build attractive confederate expressed greater body dissatisfaction. With regard to media influences, research has focused on gaining a better understanding of moderating and mediating factors. Appearance anxiety following exposure to idealized female images has been found to be greater for high self-objectifiers (Monro and Huon 2005), while self-esteem moderates the impact of attractiveness comparisons with idealized images (Jones and Buckingham 2005). Self-improvement objectives compared with self-evaluation motives for body comparisons have also been shown to have different impacts on body image (Halliwell and Dittmar 2005). Finally, a media literacy intervention prior to exposure to idealized female images was found to prevent the adverse effect of exposure (Yamamiya *et al.* 2005).

Male body image

With the increasing emphasis on the 'ideal' masculine body, there has been a corresponding increase in the amount of research focusing on male body dissatisfaction. Comparisons have been made between body image in men from different cultures (Yang *et al.* 2005) and men with different sexual orientations (Kaminski *et al.* 2005; Kimmel and Mahalik 2005; Levesque and Vichesky 2006; Reilly and Rudd 2006). Moving from descriptive studies, Jones and Crawford (2005) evaluated a dual pathway model for body dissatisfaction in adolescent boys, finding empirical support for the importance of distinguishing between muscularity and weight concerns in the development of male concerns about body image.

Negative impact of poor body image

Recent research has highlighted associations between body dissatisfaction, health risk behaviors, disordered eating and general psychopathology. Body dissatisfaction has been shown to be correlated with risky sexual behavior (Littleton *et al.* 2005b; Gillen *et al.* 2006), substance abuse (Nieri *et al.* 2005), smoking (Clark *et al.* 2005) and smoking cessation attempts (Dobmeyer *et al.* 2005; King *et al.* 2005). More compelling evidence for the negative impact of body dissatisfaction is provided by longitudinal studies examining body dissatisfaction as a predictor of outcomes after controlling for initial body dissatisfaction. In a five-year follow-up study of adolescents, body dissatisfaction has been observed to predict the development of higher levels of dieting, unhealthy and very unhealthy weight loss behaviors and binge eating, lower levels of physical activity (Neumark-Sztainer *et al.* 2006b), and low self-esteem and depressive symptoms (Paxton *et al.* 2006b). A 10-month follow-up study of 13–15 year old girls revealed that body dissatisfaction was a prospective risk factor for abnormal eating attitudes, bulimic symptoms, emotional eating, stress, low self-esteem and depression (Johnson and Wardle 2005). Analyses indicated that body dissatisfaction rather than dietary restraint was a key risk factor for this symptomatology. Tiggemann (2005b) observed that poor body image predicted low self-esteem in adolescent girls over a one-year follow-up period. Finally, Rodriguez-Cano *et al.* (2006) followed early adolescents over two years and found that body dissatisfaction prospectively predicted suicide attempts. Thus research from 2005 and 2006 has provided strong evidence that body dissatisfaction has broad negative consequences in both boys and girls.

Intervention for body dissatisfaction

Prevention in children and adolescents

Evaluations of school-based primary prevention curricula have continued, reflecting recognition that school environments are both critical social environments for the development of body image, and also environments in which many children can readily be reached, preferably prior to the onset of high levels of body dissatisfaction. Greater attention than before has been given to improving body satisfaction in children rather than in adolescents. In children, mixed results have been reported. Decreases in body dissatisfaction have been observed following a 10-session primary prevention intervention with fifth-grade girls, based on identified risk and protective factors (Scime *et al.* 2006), and following a 12-session curriculum-based primary prevention program piloted with 8–12 year old girls (DeBate and Thompson 2005). However, an eight-session physical activity intervention in children from grades three to six had no impact on body dissatisfaction in either girls or boys (McCabe *et al.* 2006).

Curricula for adolescent girls continue to be explored. On the principle that media internalization has been shown to be a causal risk factor for body dissatisfaction and disordered eating, Wilksch *et al.* (2006) examined the impact of the first phase of an interactive school-based media literacy curriculum designed to reduce media internalization in early adolescents. They observed that it was valuable to include boys in the intervention program. Statistically, boys appeared to benefit more from the media literacy lesson than girls did. However, the clinical difference was not pronounced. Although school-based prevention programs frequently have short-term effects, curriculum content is likely to need further refinement to enhance their effectiveness (Durkin *et al.* 2005), and many serious challenges remain (Neumark-Sztainer *et al.* 2006a).

Targeted interventions for high-risk women

Interventions for young women who have clear precursors of eating disorders, known as 'targeted' interventions, continue to demonstrate positive body image outcomes over extended follow-up periods. Computer-delivered psycho-educational programs appear to be particularly effective in this group. Franko *et al.* (2005) found that the interactive CD-ROM, *Food, Mood and Attitude*, reduced shape and weight concerns in high-risk college women. A further important study examined the effect of the asynchronous Internet-based computer program, *Student Bodies*, on weight and shape concerns in a large sample of college women at risk for developing eating disorders (Taylor *et al.* 2006). The authors found that the program significantly reduced weight and shape concerns compared with the control, and these changes were maintained for up to two years. Dissonance-based programs (Roehrig *et al.* 2006) and psycho-educational programs (Stice *et al.* 2006) have also been shown to reduce body dissatisfaction in targeted interventions.

Treatment of body dissatisfaction in clinical disorders

With growing appreciation of the negative implications of body dissatisfaction, with or without eating pathology, closer examination of body image intervention techniques, delivery modes and delivery settings is taking place. Delinsky and Wilson (2006) have shown that mirror exposure significantly improved body checking and avoidance, and weight and shape concerns, compared with a non-directive therapy. Gollings and Paxton (2006) reported reductions in body dissatisfaction of a large effect size following a cognitive–behavioral, therapist-led, body image intervention program delivered either face to face or via a synchronous Internet chat-room. Nye and Cash (2006) demonstrated that a group cognitive–behavioral body image program based on *The Body Image Workbook* (Cash 1997) reduced body image concerns in a clinical population of women with a range of eating disorder diagnoses who were being treated in the context of 'usual care' in a private practice. Finally, Jarry and Ip (2005) conducted an informative meta-analysis of cognitive–behavioral interventions for body image disturbance and, among other conclusions, found that behavioral rather than investment dimensions of body image improved the most, clinical samples improved more than college samples, and therapist-assisted therapy was more effective than self-directed therapy.

Summary of important findings and clinical implications

For many girls and boys, body image concerns start in primary school, and increase during adolescence. They are now recognized as problems that affect individuals in different cultures around the world. Body dissatisfaction appears to be increasing over time, although in some countries this change may be partly attributable to increases in BMI. To enhance body image research, a large number of new assessment instruments have been developed, including measures to assess positive and negative verbal commentary about appearance, body appreciation, gender- and culture-appropriate measures, and body image coping strategies.

There have been particularly important developments in relation to understanding psychosocial risk factors for body dissatisfaction in children. Studies suggest that sociocultural influences, including peer desire for thinness, exposure to media which has an emphasis on appearance and the thin ideal and exposure to dolls such as Barbie, are risk factors for body dissatisfaction at particular life stages. In adolescence, both social factors (friend dieting and weight teasing) and psychological factors (low self-esteem and depressive symptoms) have been identified as increasing the risk of development of body dissatisfaction. In women but not in men, body dissatisfaction has also been found to show moderate to high heritability.

Recent research has provided strong support for the negative impact of body dissatisfaction, not only by increasing the risk of eating disorders but also by increasing the risk of depressive symptoms and low self-esteem. In the light of this negative impact of body dissatisfaction, there has been continued focus on evaluating selective prevention interventions, but these have met with mixed results. Importantly, research indicates that targeted interventions, including those using Internet technologies, have considerable promise. Within clinical settings, cognitive–behavioral body image interventions contribute to large improvements in body image.

Future directions

Although the prevalence of body dissatisfaction (frequently defined as a desire to change some aspect of one's physical appearance, such as size) has been identified in numerous samples, in order to fully understand the epidemiology of body image problems it will be necessary to clarify the extent to which body dissatisfaction causes psychosocial distress, rather than simply a cognitive desire to be physically different. In addition, a greater understanding of body image prevalence, phenomenology, and risk factors in groups other than girls and young women in western and non-western countries is required.

The impact of psychological attributes and social–environmental factors on body dissatisfaction has been clarified in recent years. Although there is room for further understanding in this area, identification of ways to modify these risk factors so as to successfully prevent the development of body dissatisfaction remains the greatest challenge in the field. Although targeted interventions are increasingly being shown to be very valuable, and will clearly remain necessary, it may be argued that they are essentially too late. Ways of empowering girls and boys to manage the constant bombardment with social and media messages that have a negative impact on body image have yet to be perfected for any developmental stage. Too few strategies for changing social environments that contribute to body dissatisfaction have been developed or systematically evaluated. In addition, in an era that is concerned about the negative health implications of high BMI and the increasing prevalence of obesity in children and adults, a further research challenge is to successfully integrate healthy body image, eating and activity interventions. Despite the distance that we still have to travel in this regard, this review highlights the energy in the field and the extensive groundwork that has been established for future research.

References

(References included from the targeted review years are preceded by one asterisk. References preceded by three asterisks are of particular significance. The significance is explained by a short commentary following the complete reference.)

*Al-Adawi S, Dorvlo ASS, Martin RG, Yoishiuchi K, Kumano H and Kuboki T (2006) Cultural differences in Western, Indian and Omani adolescents to eating, weight and body image attitudes. In: Swain PI, editor. *New Developments in Eating Disorders Research.* Hauppauge, NY: Nova Science Publishers.

*Avalos L, Tylka TL and Wood-Barcalow N (2005) The Body Appreciation Scale: development and psychometric evaluation. *Body Image,* **2:** 285–97.

*Bearman SK, Presnell K, Martinez E and Stice E (2006) The skinny on body dissatisfaction: a longitudinal study of adolescent girls and boys. *Journal of Youth and Adolescence,* **35:** 229–41.

*Becker AE, Gilman SE and Burwell RA (2005) Changes in prevalence of overweight and in body image among Fijian women between 1989 and 1998. *Obesity Research,* **13:** 110–17.

*Britton LE, Martz DM, Bazzini DG, Curtin LA and LeaShomb A (2006) Fat talk and self-presentation of body image: is there a social norm for women to self-degrade? *Body Image,* **3:** 247–54.

*Cafri G, Yamamiya Y, Brannick M and Thompson JK (2005) The influence of sociocultural factors on body image: a meta-analysis. *International Journal of Eating Disorders,* **37:** 150–55.

Cash TF (1997) *The Body Image Workbook: an 8-step program for learning to like your looks.* Oakland, CA: New Harbinger.

*Cash TF, Santos MT and Williams EF (2005) Coping with body-image threats and challenges: validation of the Body Image Coping Strategies Inventory. *Journal of Psychosomatic Research,* **58:** 191–9.

*Chen H, Jackson T and Huang X (2006) The Negative Physical Self Scale: initial development and validation in samples of Chinese adolescents and young adults. *Body Image,* **3:** 401–12.

*Clark L and Tiggemann M (2006) Appearance culture in 9- to 12-year-old girls: media and peer influence on body dissatisfaction. *Social Development,* **15:** 628–43.

*Clark MM, Croghan IT, Reading S, Schroeder DR, Stoner SM, Patten CA *et al.* (2005) The relationship of body image dissatisfaction to cigarette smoking in college students. *Body Image,* **2:** 263–70.

*Cuzzolaro M, Vetrone G, Marano G and Garfinkel PE (2006) The Body Uneasiness Test (BUT): development and validation of a new body image assessment scale. *Eating and Weight Disorders,* **11:** 1–13.

*DeBate RD and Thompson SH (2005) Girls on the run: improvements in self-esteem, body size satisfaction and eating attitudes/behaviors. *Eating and Weight Disorders,* **10:** 25–32.

*Delinsky SS and Wilson GT (2006) Mirror exposure for the treatment of body image disturbance. *International Journal of Eating Disorders,* **39:** 108–16.

***Dittmar H, Halliwell E and Ive S (2006) Does Barbie make girls want to be thin? The effects of experimental exposure to images on the body image of 5- to 8-year-old girls. *Developmental Psychology,* **42:** 283–92.

This experimental study examined the impact of images of a Barbie doll, an Emme doll (a US size 16) and neutral pictures on body image in young girls. After exposure to images of a Barbie doll, but not an Emme doll or neutral images, the younger girls, but not the older ones, expressed heightened body dissatisfaction. These findings suggest that viewing Barbie dolls in particular has a direct impact on young girls' body image, and that there are some ages at which girls are particularly susceptible to Barbie as an aspirational role model.

*Dobmeyer AC, Peterson AL, Runyan CR, Hunter CM and Blackman LR (2005) Body image and tobacco cessation: relationships with weight concerns and intention to resume tobacco use. *Body Image,* **2:** 187–92.

*Dohnt HK and Tiggemann M (2006a) Body image concerns in young girls: the role of peers and media prior to adolescence. *Journal of Youth and Adolescence,* **35:** 141–51.

***Dohnt H and Tiggemann M (2006b) The contribution of peer and media influences to the development of body satisfaction and self-esteem in young girls: a prospective study. *Developmental Psychology*, **42**: 929–36.

This prospective study examined appearance satisfaction in 5–8 year old girls (Time 1) and again one year later (Time 2). It found that perceived peer desire for thinness and appearance television exposure (i.e. exposure to media which has an emphasis on appearance) negatively predicted appearance satisfaction at Time 2 after controlling for appearance satisfaction at Time 1. The authors concluded that young girls live in a culture in which peers and the media constantly communicate the importance of the thin ideal, which has a negative impact on their body image and self-esteem.

*Durkin S, Paxton SJ and Wertheim EH (2005) How do adolescent girls evaluate body dissatisfaction prevention messages? *Journal of Adolescent Health*, **37**: 381–90.

*Eisenberg ME, Neumark-Sztainer D and Paxton SJ (2006) Five-year change in body satisfaction among adolescents. *Journal of Psychosomatic Research*, **61**: 521–7.

***Franko DL, Mintz LB, Villapiano M, Green TC, Mainelli D *et al.* (2005) *Food, Mood and Attitude*: reducing risk for eating disorders in college women. *Health Psychology*, **24**: 567–78.

This study evaluated the new CD-ROM prevention program, Food, Mood and Attitude, in college women. The program improved all outcome measures compared with controls, but significant three-way interactions demonstrated that at-risk participants in the intervention group improved to a greater extent than the low-risk participants.

*Gillen MM, Lefkowitz ES and Shearer CL (2006) Does body image play a role in risky sexual behavior and attitudes? *Journal of Youth and Adolescence*, **35**: 243–55.

*Gollings EK and Paxton SJ (2006) Comparison of Internet and face-to-face delivery of a group body image and disordered eating intervention for women: a pilot study. *Eating Disorders*, **14**: 1–15.

*Grabe S and Hyde JS (2006) Ethnicity and body dissatisfaction among women in the United States: a meta-analysis. *Psychological Bulletin*, **132**: 622–40.

*Halliwell E and Dittmar H (2005) The role of self-improvement and self-evaluation motives in social comparisons with idealized female bodies in the media. *Body Image*, **2**: 249–61.

*Herbozo S and Thompson JK (2006) Development and validation of the Verbal Commentary on Physical Appearance Scale: considering both positive and negative commentary. *Body Image*, **3**: 255–62.

*Jakatdar TA, Cash TF and Engle EK (2006) Body-image thought processes: the development and initial validation of the Assessment of Body-Image Cognitive Distortions. *Body Image*, **3**: 325–33.

***Jarry JL and Ip K (2005) The effectiveness of stand-alone cognitive–behavioral therapy for body image: a meta-analysis. *Body Image*, **2**: 317–31.

This meta-analysis of cognitive–behavioral interventions for body image disturbance provides support for body image interventions. The authors found that behavioral rather than investment dimensions of body image improved the most, clinical samples improved more than college students, and therapist-assisted therapy was more effective than self-directed therapy.

*Johnson F and Wardle J (2005) Dietary restraint, body dissatisfaction and psychological distress: a prospective analysis. *Journal of Abnormal Psychology*, **114**: 119–25.

*Jones AM and Buckingham JT (2005) Self-esteem as a moderator of the effect of social comparison on women's body image. *Journal of Social and Clinical Psychology*, **24**: 1164–87.

*Jones DC and Crawford JK (2005) Adolescent boys and body image: weight and muscularity concerns as dual pathways to body dissatisfaction. *Journal of Youth and Adolescence*, **34**: 629–36.

*Jung J and Lee S (2006) Cross-cultural comparisons of appearance self-schema, body image, self-esteem and dieting behaviour between Korean and U.S. women. *Family and Consumer Sciences Research Journal*, **34**: 350–65.

*Kaminski PL, Chapman BP, Haynes SD and Own L (2005) Body image, eating behaviors and attitudes toward exercise among gay and straight men. *Eating Behaviors*, **6**: 179–87.

*Kelly AM, Wall M, Eisenberg ME, Story M and Neumark-Sztainer D (2005) Adolescent girls with high body satisfaction: who are they and what can they teach us? *Journal of Adolescent Health*, **37**: 391–6.

*Keski-Rahkonen A, Bulik CM, Neale BM, Rose RJ, Rissanen A and Kaprio J (2005) Body dissatisfaction and drive for thinness in young adult twins. *International Journal of Eating Disorders*, **37**: 188–99.

*Kimmel SB and Mahalik JR (2005) Body image concerns of gay men: the role of minority stress and conformity to masculine norms. *Journal of Consulting and Clinical Psychology*, **73**: 1185–90.

*King TK, Matacin M, White KS and Marcus BH (2005) A prospective examination of body image and smoking cessation in women. *Body Image*, **2**: 19–28.

*Krones PG, Stice E, Batres C and Orjada K (2005) *In vivo* social comparison to a thin-ideal peer promotes body dissatisfaction: a randomized experiment. *International Journal of Eating Disorders*, **38**: 134–42.

*Levesque MJ and Vichesky DR (2006) Raising the bar on the body beautiful: an analysis of the body image concerns of homosexual men. *Body Image*, **3**: 45–55.

*Li Y, Hu K, Ma W, Wu J and Ma G (2005) Body image perceptions among Chinese children and adolescents. *Body Image*, **2**: 91–103.

*Littleton HL, Axsom D and Pury CS (2005a) Development of the Body Image Concern Inventory. *Behaviour Research and Therapy*, **43**: 229–41.

*Littleton H, Breitkopf CR and Berenson A (2005b) Body image and risk sexual behaviors: an investigation in a tri-ethnic sample. *Body Image*, **2**: 193–8.

*Lunde C, Frisén A and Hwang CP (2006) Is peer victimization related to body esteem in 10-year-old girls and boys? *Body Image*, **3**: 25–33.

*McArthur LH, Holbert D and Peña M (2005) An exploration of the attitudinal and perceptual dimension of body image among male and female adolescents from six Latin American cities. *Adolescence*, **40**: 801–16.

McCabe MP, Ricciardelli LA and Salmon J (2006) Evaluation of a prevention program to address body focus and negative affect among children. *Journal of Health Psychology*, **11**: 589–98.

*Mangweth-Matzek B, Rupp CI, Hausmann A, Assmayr K, Mariacher E, Kemmler G *et al.* (2006) Never too old for eating disorders or body dissatisfaction: a community study of elderly women. *International Journal of Eating Disorders*, **39**: 583–6.

*Monro F and Huon G (2005) Media-portrayed idealized images, body shame, and appearance anxiety. *International Journal of Eating Disorders*, **38**: 85–90.

*Neumark-Sztainer D, Levine M, Paxton S, Smolak L, Piran N and Wertheim E (2006a) Prevention of body dissatisfaction and disordered eating: what next? *Eating Disorders: Journal of Treatment and Prevention*, **14**: 265–85.

*Neumark-Sztainer D, Paxton SJ, Hannan PJ, Haines J and Story M (2006b) Does body satisfaction matter? Five-year longitudinal associations between body satisfaction and health behaviors in adolescent females and males. *Journal of Adolescent Health*, **39**: 244–51.

*Newman DL, Sontag LM and Salvato R (2006) Psychosocial aspects of body mass and body image among rural American and Indian adolescents. *Journal of Youth and Adolescence*, **35**: 281–91.

*Nieri T, Kulis S, Keith VM and Hurdle D (2005) Body image, acculturation and substance abuse among boys and girls in the Southwest. *American Journal of Drug and Alcohol Abuse*, **31:** 617–39.

*Nye S and Cash TF (2006) Outcomes of manualized cognitive-behavioral body image therapy with eating-disordered women treated in a private clinical practice. *Eating Disorders: Journal of Treatment and Prevention*, **14:** 31–40.

*Osman A, Barrios FX, Kopper BA, Gutierrez PM, Williams JE and Bailey J (2006) The Body Influence Assessment Inventory (BIAI): development and initial validation. *Journal of Clinical Psychology*, **62:** 923–42.

*Paxton SJ, Norris M, Wertheim EH, Durkin SJ and Anderson J (2005) Body dissatisfaction, dating, and importance of thinness to attractiveness in adolescent girls. *Sex Roles*, **53:** 663–75.

***Paxton SJ, Eisenberg ME and Neumark-Sztainer D (2006a) Prospective predictors of body dissatisfaction in adolescent girls and boys: a five-year longitudinal study. *Developmental Psychology*, **42:** 888–99.

In a prospective study with a 5-year follow-up, Time 1 BMI, friend dieting and low self-esteem in early adolescent girls, BMI, socioeconomic status (SES) and weight teasing in early adolescent boys, BMI, SES and low self-esteem in middle adolescent girls, and BMI, ethnicity and depression in middle adolescent boys were found to be risk factors for Time 2 body dissatisfaction, after controlling for Time 1 body dissatisfaction.

*Paxton SJ, Neumark-Sztainer D, Hannan PJ and Eisenberg M (2006b) Body dissatisfaction prospectively predicts depressive symptoms and low self-esteem in adolescent girls and boys. *Journal of Clinical Child and Adolescent Psychology*, **35:** 539–49.

*Rasnake LK, Laube E, Lewis M and Linscheid TR (2005) Children's nutritional judgments: relation to eating attitudes and body image. *Health Communication*, **18:** 275–89.

*Reilly A and Rudd NA (2006) Is internalized homonegativity related to body image? *Family and Consumer Sciences Research Journal*, **35:** 58–73.

*Ricciardelli LA, McCabe MP, Lillis J and Thomas K (2006) A longitudinal investigation of the development of weight and muscle concerns among preadolescent boys. *Journal of Youth and Adolescence*, **35:** 177–87.

*Rodriguez-Cano T, Beato-Fernandez L and Llario AB (2006) Body dissatisfaction as a predictor of self-reported suicide attempts in adolescents: a Spanish community prospective study. *Journal of Adolescent Health*, **38:** 684–8.

*Roehrig M, Thompson JK, Brannick M and van den Berg P (2006) Dissonance-based eating disorder prevention program: a preliminary dismantling investigation. *International Journal of Eating Disorders*, **39:** 1–10.

*Scime M, Cook-Cottone C, Kane L and Watson T (2006) Group prevention of eating disorders with fifth-grade females: impact on body dissatisfaction, drive for thinness, and media influence. *Eating Disorders: Journal of Treatment and Prevention*, **14:** 143–55.

*Shroff H and Thompson JK (2006) The tripartite influence model of body image and eating disturbance: a replication with adolescent girls. *Body Image*, **3:** 17–23.

*Siervo M, Grey P, Nyan OA and Prentice AM (2006) A pilot study on body image, attractiveness and body size in Gambians living in an urban community. *Eating and Weight Disorders*, **11:** 100–9.

*Sim L and Zeman J (2006) The contribution of emotion regulation to body dissatisfaction and disordered eating in early adolescent girls. *Journal of Youth and Adolescence*, **35:** 219–28.

*Smolak L and Stein JA (2006) The relationship of drive for muscularity to sociocultural factors, self-esteem, physical attributes, gender role and social comparison in middle school boys. *Body Image*, **3:** 121–9.

*Stanford JN and McCabe MP (2005) Evaluation of a body image prevention programme for adolescent boys. *European Eating Disorders Review*, **13**: 360–70.

*Stice E, Orjada K and Tristan J (2006) Trial of a psychoeducational eating disturbance intervention for college women: a replication and extension. *International Journal of Eating Disorders*, **39**: 233–9.

*Storvoll EE, Strandbu A and Wichstrom L (2005) A cross-sectional study of changes in Norwegian adolescents' body image from 1992 to 2002. *Body Image*, **2**: 5–18.

*Taylor BC, Bryson S, Luce KH, Cunning D, Doyle AC, Abascal LB *et al.* (2006) Prevention of eating disorders in at-risk college-age women. *Archives of General Psychiatry*, **63**: 881–8.

*Tiggemann M (2005a) The role of media exposure in adolescent girls' body dissatisfaction and drive for thinness: prospective results. *Journal of Social and Clinical Psychology*, **25**: 523–41.

*Tiggemann M (2005b) Body dissatisfaction and adolescent self-esteem: prospective findings. *Body Image*, **2**: 129–35.

*Toro J, Castro J, Gila A and Pombo C (2005) Assessment of sociocultural influences on the body shape model in adolescent males with anorexia nervosa. *European Eating Disorders Review*, **13**: 351–9.

*Tylka TL, Bergeron D and Schwartz JP (2005) Development and psychometric evaluation of the Male Body Attitudes Scale (MBAS). *Body Image: an International Journal of Research*, **2**: 161–75.

*White MA and Grilo CA (2005) Ethnic differences in the prediction of eating and body image disturbances among female adolescent psychiatric inpatients. *International Journal of Eating Disorders*, **38**: 78–84.

*Wilksch SM, Tiggemann M and Wade T (2006) Impact of interactive school-based media literacy lessons for reducing internalization of media ideals in young adolescent girls and boys. *International Journal of Eating Disorders*, **39**: 385–93.

*Wojtowicz AE and von Ranson KM (2006) Psychometric evaluation of two scales examining muscularity concerns in men and women. *Psychology of Men and Masculinity*, **7**: 56–66.

*Yamamiya Y, Cash TF, Melnyk SE, Posavac HD and Posavac SS (2005) Women's exposure to thin-and-beautiful media images: body image effects of media-ideal internalization and impact-reduction interventions. *Body Image*, **2**: 74–80.

*Yang CJ, Gray P and Pope HG Jr (2005) Male body image in Taiwan versus the West: Yanggang Zhiqi meets the Adonis complex. *American Journal of Psychiatry*, **162**: 263–9.

6

Personality and eating disorders

Kristin M von Ranson

Abstract

Objectives of review. This chapter reviews research findings from 2005 and 2006 regarding dimensional personality traits, categorical personality disorders and dimensional personality pathology, and categorical personality subtypes in eating disorders.

Summary of recent findings. Approaches linking specific personality traits to eating pathology have demonstrated the predictive validity of perfectionism and impulsiveness. Impulsive behaviors are associated with compulsivity and purging behaviors, and may occur in individuals with restricting anorexia nervosa despite contradictory self-reports. Personality pathology is common among patients with eating disorders. Individuals in the community who have a personality disorder by early adulthood are at increased risk of developing an eating disorder. Several recent studies have supported a three-cluster personality typology across eating disorders, consisting of resilient/high-functioning, undercontrolled/emotionally dysregulated and overcontrolled/constricted types.

Future directions. Future research using community samples, that attempts to explicate and replicate the three-cluster personality typology, and pays close attention to methodological issues and generalizability of findings, is recommended.

Introduction

Why do some people develop eating disorders (EDs) when many or most of their peers do not? Are there ways to predict who is at elevated risk for eating pathology before the onset of symptoms? What individual-level factors influence the symptoms, course and duration of EDs? Personality traits – enduring characteristics that define important aspects of who we are – are postulated to play a causal role in the etiology, symptomatic expression and maintenance of ED symptoms. Similarly, personality disorders, which involve maladaptive personality traits (American Psychiatric Association 1994), are frequently found among patients and community members with EDs (Cassin and von Ranson 2005). Not only do major theories of EDs suppose that personality factors are diatheses for eating pathology, but also prospective research has found that personality variables have predictive value for ED symptoms (e.g. Leon *et al.* 1999).

The study of personality in EDs is fraught with methodological complexity due to several measurement issues, including the use of a range of measures with distinct definitions of personality dimensions, the problem of separating lasting personality traits from shorter-lived states that are impacted by starvation and active Axis I psychopathology, and the frequent reliance upon clinical samples, which may present a biased picture of personality (for a detailed discussion, see Cassin and von Ranson 2005; Vitousek and Stumpf 2005; Lilenfeld *et al.* 2006). Taxometric issues, or issues related to classification, further complicate the study of personality in EDs, including the temporal instability of ED subtypes over time (e.g. Eddy *et al.* 2002), whereas personality characteristics are presumed to be temporally stable.

Accordingly, the research literature on personality and EDs is characterized by inconsistencies as well as trends. Many attempts have been made to link ED symptoms to specific personality types, but few personality factors have been consistently shown to discriminate between ED diagnoses, in part because of the personality heterogeneity within and between diagnoses. Personality variables linked to both anorexia nervosa (AN) and bulimia nervosa (BN) include perfectionism, obsessive-compulsiveness, neuroticism, negative emotionality, harm avoidance, low self-directedness, low cooperativeness, and avoidant personality disorder traits (Cassin and von Ranson 2005). Individuals with restricting anorexia nervosa (ANR) are often characterized by high levels of constraint and persistence and low levels of novelty seeking, whereas individuals with bulimic symptoms of binge eating or purging often show high levels of impulsiveness, sensation seeking and novelty seeking (Cassin and von Ranson 2005). However, although these descriptors fit a large percentage of people with EDs, many exceptions remain, thus limiting the utility of this trait–ED symptom matching approach (Steiger and Bruce 2004).

If ED symptoms are not consistently associated with particular personality types, how else might we conceptualize the role of personality in EDs? In recent years, researchers have begun to pay attention to the heterogeneity of personality characteristics across ED diagnoses, shifting their focus to personality subtypes describing the broad array of ED diagnoses, rather than types specific to AN, BN or eating disorder not otherwise specified (EDNOS) individually. Data analytic approaches that identify latent taxons in personality data have been used to identify ED subtypes (e.g. Bulik *et al.* 2000; Westen and Harnden-Fischer 2001; Wade *et al.* 2006).

Literature review

This chapter will review the findings of recent English-language studies (published in 2005 or 2006) which have used one of three general approaches to the conceptualization of personality in EDs, namely personality traits, Axis II personality disorders, and personality subtypes. It will then discuss the clinical implications of recent research, and future directions for research.

Personality traits

Empirical studies of personality traits – that is, dimensional personality variations that describe individuals' typical ways of thinking, acting and feeling – tend to describe either specific traits that have been observed in clinical samples of individuals with EDs, or profiles on normal-range, comprehensive personality inventories. Perfectionism, impulsiveness and obsessive-compulsiveness are among the most commonly researched personality traits in EDs.

Perfectionism

Perfectionism is commonly found in individuals with AN, BN and binge-eating disorder (BED) (Cassin and von Ranson 2005). A combination of perfectionism, perceived weight status and self-efficacy was shown to prospectively predict the development of binge eating among 406 university women (Bardone-Cone *et al.* 2006), suggesting that perfectionism plays a key role in the development of eating pathology.

Perfectionism has increasingly been viewed as a multifactorial construct. A recent factor analysis of 286 university women identified three factors of the perfectionism construct, namely normal perfectionism, neurotic perfectionism, and orderliness (Pearson and Gleaves 2006). Neurotic perfectionism was strongly associated with bulimic symptoms, body dissatisfaction and self-esteem. Neurotic perfectionism was so highly correlated with self-esteem ($r = -0.92$) in this sample that these constructs may be essentially identical.

A semi-structured interview was developed to retrospectively evaluate pre-morbid personality traits among 85 teenage girls and 14 teenage boys who were receiving treatment for AN (Strober *et al.* 2006). Researchers found high levels of perfectionism (in 72.9% of females and 50% of males) and no gender differences. Psychometric data on the interview are lacking.

Perfectionism, particularly concern about mistakes, has been linked to obsessive-compulsive features of obsessive-compulsive disorder (OCD) or obsessive-compulsive personality disorder (OCPD). A study of 607 individuals with EDs found similar rates of OCD and OCPD across ED subtypes, and found the highest levels of perfectionism in individuals with OCPD (Halmi *et al.* 2005). Perfectionistic concern about mistakes and doubts about actions were especially closely linked to OCPD in this sample. Other research investigating associations between perfectionism and EDs among 1119 postpartum women reported that concern about mistakes or a history of an ED were associated with elevated risk for postpartum depression (Mazzeo *et al.* 2006). Concern about mistakes was also associated with ED symptoms in a study of 145 high school girls (Sassaroli and Ruggiero 2005).

Impulsiveness

A number of recent studies have addressed the relationship of impulsiveness to ED diagnoses and symptoms. Consistent with previous findings (Cassin and von Ranson 2005), one study reported that impulsiveness was associated with poor 12-year outcome from AN (Fichter *et al.* 2006).

Findings from a study which assessed impulsive behaviors, rather than propensity toward impulsiveness, suggested that impulsive behaviors were associated with purging but not with binge eating. A study of 554 patients with EDs (183 patients with ANR and 65 with binge-eating/purging anorexia nervosa (ANBP); 244 patients with purging type BN (BNP) and 62 with non-purging type BN) found that about half of the sample reported at least one type of impulsive behavior, 35% reported more than one, and 13% reported more than three (Favaro *et al.* 2005). Individuals with impulsive behaviors tended to exhibit personality characteristics of high novelty seeking and low persistence. These authors observed that impulsive behaviors were linked to more severe psychopathology and ED symptoms.

To test the theory that four personality traits – urgency, low perseverance, low premeditation, and sensation seeking ('UPPS') – form different pathways to impulsive behavior, Claes *et al.* (2005) evaluated 146 female ED inpatients. Patients with ANR reported less impulsiveness on the four UPPS personality traits than patients with ANBP or BNP. Impulsiveness may underlie both bulimic symptoms in ANBP and BN and other 'multi-impulsive' behaviors, such as substance abuse and self-injurious behavior. Consistent with this interpretation, women with BED and comorbid lifetime substance use disorder reported more impulsiveness than women with BED but no lifetime substance use disorder (Peterson *et al.* 2005).

Some research reports focusing on impulsiveness among individuals with EDs have begun to cast doubt on the conventional wisdom that impulsiveness primarily affects individuals with bulimic symptoms (Cassin and von Ranson 2005). Individuals with ANR may lack insight into their impulsive behaviors, and thus impulsiveness in AN may be more complex than was previously thought. For example, whereas patients with ANR self-reported low levels of impulsiveness compared with controls and patients with purging AN or BN, their performance on behavioral tasks documented a conflicting lack of inhibitory control, which was interpreted as behavioral impulsiveness (Claes *et al.* 2006a). Other research has shown that, compared with a normal control group, inpatients with AN responded rapidly but inaccurately to a continuous performance task, indicating behavioral impulsiveness, again in contrast to their low self-reported impulsiveness (Butler and Montgomery 2005). However, the latter study did not identify subtypes among the participants with AN.

Other findings have not provided clear support for the theory that individuals with AN may act more impulsively than they self-report. Although research comparing ED outpatients with non-clinical controls found increased error on a behavioral task in individuals with ANBP, and elevated self-reported cognitive impulsiveness across AN and BN diagnoses, it found elevated self-reported motor impulsiveness among individuals with bulimic symptoms only (Rosval *et al.* 2006).

Both impulsiveness and compulsivity are commonly found in individuals with EDs (Cassin and von Ranson 2005). Whereas some authors have postulated that impulsiveness and compulsivity lie at either end of a single continuum (e.g. Claes *et al.* 2005), other evidence suggests that dimensions of impulsiveness and compulsivity are distinct. A multi-site study of 204 women with BN found much variability in impulsiveness and compulsivity levels between individuals, and reported that impulsiveness and compulsivity were moderately positively correlated ($r = 0.33$), suggesting that impulsiveness and compulsivity are not poles of a single continuum (Engel *et al.* 2005). Consistent with other findings (Favaro *et al.* 2005), Engel *et al.* reported that higher levels of impulsiveness and compulsivity were associated with more impairment with regard to personality, drug and alcohol use, eating disturbances and depression. These findings are consistent with the theory that serotonin dysfunction underlies both impulsiveness and compulsivity, although longitudinal or experimental data are needed to test this theory.

The results of positron emission tomography (PET) research provided stronger evidence that serotonergic function remained altered after recovery from ANR ($n = 13$) and ANBP ($n = 12$), compared with healthy control women ($n = 18$) (Bailer *et al.* 2005). In addition, obsessive-compulsive symptoms among women with ANBP were more elevated than those of controls.

Comprehensive personality inventory and other results

Numerous recent studies show that neuroticism, or propensity towards experiencing negative emotions, is strongly associated with EDs, although its specificity to EDs is unclear. Premorbidly assessed neuroticism predicted the subsequent development of AN in a population-based sample of 31 406 Swedish twins (Bulik *et al.* 2006). Recent results involving the Eysenck Personality Questionnaire suggest that the interaction of neuroticism and introversion is correlated with eating pathology among female undergraduates (Miller *et al.* 2006). Compared with normal samples, low self-esteem and low self-directedness scores on the Temperament and Character Inventory were associated with poorer long-term outcome among 44 female former AN patients (Halvorsen and Heyerdahl 2006).

A study of patients with AN ($n = 14$) or BN ($n = 11$) found that women with an ED inhibited their expression of emotions more than 31 women without an ED, after controlling for neuroticism, and experienced more neuroticism and hostility (Forbush and Watson 2006). Women with an ED were also more aware of others' thoughts and expectations and less aware of their own inner thoughts and feelings than controls. The authors speculated that individuals who have difficulty identifying or expressing their emotions may turn bad feelings (e.g. feeling fat) inward. Research investigating specific emotion regulation processes, including negative emotionality, poor awareness of emotion, and non-constructive coping with negative emotion, in 234 early adolescent girls found that these variables partially mediated the relationship between body dissatisfaction and bulimic symptoms (Sim and Zeman 2005).

Studies that examined serotonergic neurotransmission in individuals with EDs have found associations with personality dimensions that are common in people with EDs, such as increased harm avoidance in those with BN (Monteleone *et al.* 2006), and low reward dependence and low harm avoidance in adolescents with AN (Rybakowski *et al.* 2006).

Personality disorders

The findings of studies of personality disorders and personality pathology, which are commonly reported in ED patients, tend to correspond to the findings of studies of dimensional personality traits (Cassin and von Ranson 2005). Three-quarters (77%) of 74 patients with chronic EDs had at least one personality disorder diagnosis at intake to an inpatient treatment program (Ro *et al.* 2005a). At two years' follow-up, 57% had at least one personality disorder. Consistent with previous findings (Cassin and von Ranson 2005), the most frequent personality disorder diagnosis in this sample was avoidant personality disorder. There was no difference in the rates of personality disorders across different types of ED (AN, BN and EDNOS). Another report on this sample indicates that personality disorder changes followed improvements in ED symptoms (Ro *et al.* 2005b).

A study of 1021 individuals with EDs reported a high prevalence of borderline personality disorder specifically among those who abused laxatives (Tozzi *et al.* 2006). A cross-sectional study that assessed 83 ill and 55 recovered women with AN found evidence of emotional dysregulation, social inhibition and compulsivity in both groups (Holliday *et al.* 2006b), which suggests that personality pathology in AN may persist over time.

A longitudinal study of 658 community-based individuals indicated that those who had a personality disorder by the age of 22 years had an elevated risk of developing an ED by the age of 33 years (Johnson *et al.* 2006). In addition, these individuals were at elevated risk for the onset of recurrent binge eating, purging, recurrent dietary restriction, and obesity by middle adulthood. Many different kinds of personality disorder symptoms (i.e. borderline, histrionic, antisocial, schizotypal and depressive) contributed to the development of eating and weight problems.

Personality subtypes

There is accumulating evidence which suggests that personality types do not correspond neatly to *Diagnostic and Statistical Manual of Mental Disorders (DSM-IV)* (American Psychiatric Association, 1994) diagnoses. Personality pathology varies substantially both within and between ED diagnoses. The findings of several recent cluster and latent profile analytic studies of ED individuals (Wonderlich *et al.* 2005; Claes *et al.* 2006b; Holliday *et al.* 2006a) were consistent with earlier findings of three personality-based subtypes of EDs, namely resilient/high functioning, undercontrolled/emotionally dysregulated and over-controlled/constricted (e.g. Westen and Harnden-Fischer 2001). A study of 145 clinicians reporting on their bulimic patients provided further support for these three types (Thompson-Brenner and Westen 2005), and another study of individuals who had recovered from AN and BN replicated the latter two subtypes (Wagner *et al.* 2006). Resilient patients tended to have the lowest number of eating and comorbid symptoms, and undercontrolled patients tended to manifest more impulsive behaviors, including alcohol and drug abuse, binge eating and purging, than overcontrolled patients (Claes *et al.* 2006b). Another study identified three types comparable to those discussed above, but formed the clusters on the basis of comorbid psychopathology, and found expected differences in personality and ED symptoms (Wonderlich *et al.* 2005). The three types have distinct patterns of adaptive functioning and treatment response, with the undercontrolled patients manifesting the longest duration of illness and the most psychiatric hospitalizations (Thompson-Brenner and Westen 2005).

This three-subtype finding appears to be robust in both AN and BN patient samples and across different types of self-reported personality data, including the Big Five personality dimensions and DSM-IV personality pathology. In addition, these three personality subtypes accommodate the finding of frequent diagnostic crossover among individuals with EDs over time, in that the three personality subtypes exist across diagnoses and do not correspond to a specific constellation of ED symptoms.

Summary of important findings

The research reported in this review supports the conclusion that the relationships between personality and EDs are quite complex, and are probably influenced by numerous methodological concerns. Specific findings of note follow. Recent research on perfectionism has illustrated its predictive utility with ED symptoms, and has highlighted its association with OCPD. A recent study has also supported the multifactorial nature of perfectionism. Major recent findings suggest that impulsiveness is associated with poor long-term treatment outcome, that impulsiveness and compulsivity appear to be orthogonal dimensions, that impulsive behaviors are associated with purging but not with binge eating, and that individuals with AN may be more impulsive than was initially thought. Personality pathology is very common among acutely ill patients with EDs. Another important recent finding was that community-based individuals who had a personality disorder by early adulthood experienced increased risk of developing an ED within a decade.

Perhaps the most intriguing and potentially important recent empirical findings with regard to personality and EDs step away from the tradition of examining one-to-one associations between personality characteristics and ED symptoms and diagnoses. Several recent studies have replicated previous findings of three personality-based clusters in ED patients, namely resilient/

high-functioning, undercontrolled/emotionally dysregulated and overcontrolled/ constricted types. Although it may be of value to continue to consider how personality traits relate to ED symptoms, it may also be fruitful to further examine the personality types that seem to underlie AN and BN. ED diagnoses tend to be temporally unstable, and therefore are limited in their ability to predict ED course or outcome. Use of personality-based subtyping acknow- ledges the personality heterogeneity that exists both within and across EDs and, if incorporated into our diagnostic system, may ultimately help to improve the predictive utility of ED diagnoses. If we capitalize on the commonalities in personality that exist in patients across specific ED diagnoses, we may be better able to predict important outcomes. Examination of these subtypes may eventually lead to the development of ED diagnoses that are less descriptive of current symptoms and possibly more reflective of underlying pathology.

Clinical implications

Comprehensive assessment of personality characteristics in ED patients is recommended, as personality variables may influence the course and sympto- matic expression of EDs. Information on personality may be useful in helping to anticipate aspects of outcome (for details, see Cassin and von Ranson 2005). For example, recent data show that impulsiveness is linked to poor treatment outcome and more psychiatric hospitalizations for EDs. For clinicians whose caseload includes individuals without EDs, it will be helpful to recall that adults with a personality disorder diagnosis are at heightened risk for developing an ED over time.

Two cautions are in order. First, it is impossible to predict any specific individual's ED outcome on the basis of research, as research describes trends and probabilities, not certainties. Secondly, awareness of the often fluid nature of personality disorders in EDs over time may enable clinicians to avoid over- interpreting the meaning of an Axis II diagnosis carried by a patient (Vitousek and Stumpf 2005). As these authors note, personality disorders are extremely common among ED patients, yet remarkably unstable over time. Data show that personality disorders in part reflect a patient's Axis I pathology, worsening when ED symptoms worsen and improving as ED symptoms improve. This principle probably applies to personality characteristics as well.

As the roles of personality traits and personality disorders in the etiology and maintenance of eating pathology continue to be studied and unravelled, these traits and symptoms may provide targets for psychotherapeutic change that may help to reduce ED symptoms (e.g. cognitive–behavioral therapy targeting clinical perfectionism, mood intolerance, low self-esteem or interpersonal dif- ficulties; Fairburn et al. 2003). The unanticipated finding of efficacy of inter- personal psychotherapy in the treatment of BN (Fairburn et al. 1993), for example, illustrates the principle that a psychotherapeutic approach need not directly address ED symptoms, but instead may have a positive impact on an ED by addressing associated problems.

Future directions

Attention to methodological issues in the study of personality and EDs is critical, as the validity of findings hinges on the methodological strength of the research conducted. This point is not unique to personality and EDs, but in such a complex area as this, it is especially important that researchers pay close attention to methodological issues when designing and carrying out studies. Thus, the following recommendations for future research emphasize specific methodological issues.

Much of the extant research on personality and EDs has involved clinical samples. Although it has long been suspected that treatment and community-based samples of individuals with EDs may differ in important respects, recent results confirmed this suspicion by illustrating that non-treatment-seeking women with AN manifested less personality pathology than treatment seekers (Perkins *et al.* 2005). This finding supports the need for more community-based, ideally epidemiological studies of personality and EDs to improve our understanding of the mechanisms that relate personality and EDs. Furthermore, attempted replications of the three personality subtypes among community-based samples of individuals with a range of EDs are needed. One aim of these replications should be to resolve key elements of the subtypes, as the subtypes that have been identified have been similar but not identical. Another issue is the need to clarify the constructs under study and reconcile the various measures used for personality constructs, as the large number of measures used contributes to difficulty in consolidating findings. Prospective research will help to clarify the temporal relationships, and thus the etiological significance, of personality in EDs. More research is needed into personality characteristics in BED samples, as well as in male individuals and ethnic minorities with EDs, to evaluate the validity of generalizing the existing findings to these groups. Finally, the use of a range of forms of assessment of personality (i.e. interviews, observational studies, behavioral assessment, and information from significant others, in addition to self-report questionnaires) will strengthen our understanding of personality phenomena and their relationship to EDs.

In conclusion, the study of personality and EDs is an exciting yet somewhat thorny area of research that has the potential to inform future treatments and prevention of EDs, as well as to help to clarify the underpinnings of eating pathology.

References

(References included from the targeted review years are preceded by one asterisk. References preceded by three asterisks are of particular significance. The significance is explained by a short commentary following the complete reference.)

American Psychiatric Association (1994) *Diagnostic and Statistical Manual of Mental Disorders* (4e). Washington, DC: American Psychiatric Association.

***Bailer UF, Frank GK, Henry SE, Price JC, Meltzer CC, Weissfeld L *et al.* (2005) Altered brain serotonin 5-HT$_{1a}$ receptor binding after recovery from anorexia nervosa measured by positron emission tomography and [^{11}C]WAY100635. *Archives of General Psychiatry,* **62:** 1032–41.

Although the sample size was small, this PET study is important because it demonstrated that altered serotonin function among former ANR patients persists after recovery and is linked to anxiety and harm avoidance, suggesting a possible neuronal basis for associations between personality and AN.

*Bardone-Cone AM, Abramson LY, Vohs KD, Heatherton TF and Joiner TE (2006) Predicting bulimic symptoms: an interactive model of self-efficacy, perfectionism, and perceived weight status. *Behaviour Research and Therapy,* **44:** 27–42.

Bulik CM, Sullivan PF and Kendler KS (2000) An empirical study of the classification of eating disorders. *American Journal of Psychiatry,* **157:** 886–95.

*Bulik CM, Sullivan PF, Tozzi F, Furberg H, Lichtenstein P and Pedersen NL (2006) Prevalence, heritability and prospective risk factors for anorexia nervosa. *Archives of General Psychiatry,* **63:** 305–12.

*Butler G and Montgomery A (2005) Subjective self-control and behavioural impulsivity coexist in anorexia nervosa. *Eating Behaviors,* **6:** 221–7.

Cassin SE and von Ranson KM (2005) Personality and eating disorders: a decade in review. *Clinical Psychology Review,* **25:** 895–916.

*Claes L, Vandereycken W and Vertommen H (2005) Impulsivity-related traits in eating disorder patients. *Personality and Individual Differences,* **39:** 739–49.

*Claes L, Nederkoorn C, Vandereycken W, Guerrieri R and Vertommen H (2006a) Impulsiveness and lack of inhibitory control in eating disorders. *Eating Behaviors,* **7:** 196–203.

***Claes L, Vandereycken W, Luyten P, Soenens B, Pieters G and Vertommen H (2006b) Personality prototypes in eating disorders based on the big five model. *Journal of Personality Disorders,* **20:** 401–16.

This study replicated a three-factor structure of personality in ED patients using a measure of normal personality dimensions. It was also the first to link this three-factor model to a similar personality typology previously described in a range of non-clinical samples, thus illustrating that this typology may be broadly descriptive of personality functioning.

Eddy KT, Keel PK, Dorer DJ, Delinsky SS, Franko DL and Herzog DB (2002) Longitudinal comparison of anorexia nervosa subtypes. *International Journal of Eating Disorders,* **31:** 191–201.

***Engel SG, Corneliussen SJ, Wonderlich SA, Crosby RD, le Grange D, Crow S *et al.* (2005) Impulsivity and compulsivity in bulimia nervosa. *International Journal of Eating Disorders,* **38:** 244–51.

This study of BN patients provided useful clarification that impulsiveness and compulsivity appear to be correlated and are not likely to be at opposite ends of the same dimension. Its strengths include the large sample size and the inclusion of data on comorbid problems, such as substance use and depression.

Fairburn CG, Jones R, Peveler RC, Hope RA and O'Connor M (1993) Psychotherapy and bulimia nervosa: longer-term effects of interpersonal psychotherapy, behavior therapy, and cognitive behavior therapy. *Archives of General Psychiatry,* **50:** 419–28.

Fairburn CG, Cooper Z and Shafran R (2003) Cognitive behaviour therapy for eating disorders: a 'transdiagnostic' theory and treatment. *Behaviour Research and Therapy,* **41:** 509–28.

*Favaro A, Zanetti T, Tenconi E, Degortes D, Ronzan A, Veronese A *et al.* (2005) The relationship between temperament and impulsive behaviors in eating disordered subjects. *Eating Disorders: the Journal of Treatment and Prevention*, **13**: 61–70.

*Fichter MM, Quadflieg N and Hedlund S (2006) Twelve-year course and outcome predictors of anorexia nervosa. *International Journal of Eating Disorders*, **39**: 87–100.

*Forbush K and Watson D (2006) Emotional inhibition and personality traits: a comparison of women with anorexia, bulimia, and normal controls. *Annals of Clinical Psychiatry*, **18**: 115–21.

*Halmi KA, Tozzi F, Thornton LM, Crow S, Fichter MM, Kaplan AS *et al.* (2005) The relation among perfectionism, obsessive-compulsive personality disorder and obsessive-compulsive disorder in individuals with eating disorders. *International Journal of Eating Disorders*, **38**: 371–4.

*Halvorsen I and Heyerdahl S (2006) Girls with anorexia nervosa as young adults: personality, self-esteem and life satisfaction. *International Journal of Eating Disorders*, **39**: 285–93.

*Holliday J, Landau S, Collier D and Treasure J (2006a) Do illness characteristics and familial risk differ between women with anorexia nervosa grouped on the basis of personality pathology? *Psychological Medicine*, **36**: 529–38.

*Holliday J, Uher R, Landau S, Collier D and Treasure J (2006b) Personality pathology among individuals with a lifetime history of anorexia nervosa. *Journal of Personality Disorders*, **20**: 417–30.

***Johnson JG, Cohen P, Kasen S and Brook JS (2006) Personality disorder traits evident by early adulthood and risk for eating and weight problems during middle adulthood. *International Journal of Eating Disorders*, **39**: 184–92.

This report described longitudinal, interview assessments of a large sample of community members at four time points, controlling for Axis I disorders. Their results linked risk for development of an ED in mid-adulthood to premorbid, adult personality disorder characteristics.

Leon GR, Fulkerson JA, Perry CL, Keel PK and Klump KL (1999) Three to four year prospective evaluation of personality and behavioral risk factors for later disordered eating in adolescent girls and boys. *Journal of Youth and Adolescence*, **28**: 181–96.

Lilenfeld LRR, Wonderlich S, Riso LP, Crosby R and Mitchell J (2006) Eating disorders and personality: a methodological and empirical review. *Clinical Psychology Review*, **26**: 299–320.

*Mazzeo SE, Landt MC, Jones I, Mitchell K, Kendler KS, Neale MC *et al.* (2006) Associations among postpartum depression, eating disorders, and perfectionism in a population-based sample of adult women. *International Journal of Eating Disorders*, **39**: 202–11.

*Miller JL, Schmidt LA, Vaillancourt T, McDougall P and Laliberte M (2006) Neuroticism and introversion: a risky combination for disordered eating among a non-clinical sample of undergraduate women. *Eating Behaviors*, **7**: 69–78.

*Monteleone P, Santonastaso P, Mauri M, Bellodi L, Erzegovesi S, Fuschino A *et al.* (2006) Investigation of the serotonin transporter regulatory region polymorphism in bulimia nervosa: relationships to harm avoidance, nutritional parameters, and psychiatric comorbidity. *Psychosomatic Medicine*, **68**: 99–103.

***Pearson CA and Gleaves DH (2006) The multiple dimensions of perfectionism and their relation with eating disorder features. *Personality and Individual Differences*, **41**: 225–35.

This study, which identified three factors within the construct of perfectionism, found strongest associations between neurotic perfectionism and bulimic symptoms, body dissatisfaction and self-esteem. These findings raise questions about the distinction between one facet of perfectionism (neurotic perfectionism) and self-esteem, which were very highly intercorrelated.

*Perkins PS, Klump KL, Iacono WG and McGue M (2005) Personality traits in women with anorexia nervosa: evidence for a treatment-seeking bias? *International Journal of Eating Disorders*, **37**: 32–7.

*Peterson CB, Miller KB, Crow SJ, Thuras P and Mitchell JE (2005) Subtypes of binge eating disorder based on psychiatric history. *International Journal of Eating Disorders*, **38**: 273–6.

*Ro O, Martinsen EW, Hoffart A and Rosenvinge J (2005a) Two-year prospective study of personality disorders in adults with longstanding eating disorders. *International Journal of Eating Disorders*, **37**: 112–18.

*Ro O, Martinsen EW, Hoffart A, Sexton H and Rosenvinge JH (2005b) The interaction of personality disorders and eating disorders: a two-year prospective study of patients with longstanding eating disorders. *International Journal of Eating Disorders*, **38**: 106–11.

*Rosval L, Steiger H, Bruce K, Israel M, Richardson J and Aubut M (2006) Impulsivity in women with eating disorders: problem of response inhibition, planning or attention? *International Journal of Eating Disorders*, **39**: 590–93.

*Rybakowski F, Slopien A, Dmitrzak-Weglarz M, Czerski P, Rajewski A and Hauser J (2006) The 5-HT2A -1438 A/G and 5-HTTLPR polymorphisms and personality dimensions in adolescent anorexia nervosa: association study. *Neuropsychobiology*, **53**: 33–9.

*Sassaroli S and Ruggiero GM (2005) The role of stress in the association between low self-esteem, perfectionism and worry, and eating disorders. *International Journal of Eating Disorders*, **37**: 135–41.

*Sim L and Zeman J (2005) Emotion regulation factors as mediators between body dissatisfaction and bulimic symptoms in early adolescent girls. *Journal of Early Adolescence*, **25**: 478–96.

Steiger H and Bruce KR (2004) Personality traits and disorders associated with anorexia nervosa, bulimia nervosa, and binge eating disorder. In: Brewerton TD, editor. *Clinical Handbook of Eating Disorders: an integrated approach. Volume 26.* New York: Marcel Dekker, pp. 209–30.

*Strober M, Freeman R, Lampert C, Diamond J, Teplinsky C and DeAntonio M (2006) Are there gender differences in core symptoms, temperament, and short-term prospective outcome in anorexia nervosa? *International Journal of Eating Disorders*, **39**: 570–75.

*Thompson-Brenner H and Westen D (2005) Personality subtypes in eating disorders: validation of a classification in a naturalistic sample. *British Journal of Psychiatry*, **186**: 516–24.

*Tozzi F, Thronton LM, Mitchell J, Fichter MM, Klump KL, Lilenfeld LR *et al.* (2006) Features associated with laxative abuse in individuals with eating disorders. *Psychosomatic Medicine*, **68**: 470–77.

Vitousek KM and Stumpf RE (2005) Difficulties in the assessment of personality traits and disorders in eating-disordered individuals. *Eating Disorders: the Journal of Treatment and Prevention*, **13**: 37–60.

*Wade TD, Crosby RD, Martin NG, Wade TD, Crosby RD and Martin NG (2006) Use of latent profile analysis to identify eating disorder phenotypes in an adult Australian twin cohort. *Archives of General Psychiatry*, **63**: 1377–84.

*Wagner A, Barbarich-Marsteller NC, Frank GK, Bailer UF, Wonderlich SA, Crosby RD *et al.* (2006) Personality traits after recovery from eating disorders: do subtypes differ? *International Journal of Eating Disorders*, **39**: 276–84.

Westen D and Harnden-Fischer J (2001) Personality profiles in eating disorders: rethinking the distinction between axis I and axis II. *American Journal of Psychiatry*, **158**: 547–62.

***Wonderlich SA, Crosby RD, Joiner T, Peterson CB, Bardone-Cone A, Klein M *et al.* (2005) Personality subtyping and bulimia nervosa: psychopathological and genetic correlates. *Psychological Medicine*, **35**: 649–57.

This article examines personality and comorbid psychopathology of a large sample of women with full criteria or subclinical BN and identifies three subtypes (affective–perfectionistic, impulsive and low comorbid psychopathology clusters). This replication supports the view that a three-factor typology of personality is useful for describing individuals with EDs.

7

Neuroimaging

Janet Treasure and Janine DesForges

Abstract

Objectives of review. This review summarizes the neuroimaging research in eating disorders published in 2005 and 2006.

Summary of recent findings. Both brain substance and basal blood flow are decreased in the acute phase of anorexia nervosa. However, it appears that these changes are reversible after recovery. In some experiments with illness-relevant cues in people with eating disorders there is less activation in the perceptual and attention networks, but greater activation in the emotional networks. An imbalance in dopamine and serotonin (5HT) receptors is present both in the acute state and after recovery in anorexia nervosa. In bulimia nervosa there are fewer opiate receptors. This is consistent with abnormalities in the reward and/or punishment (anxiety) systems.

Future directions. A new strategy may be to devise scanning experiments that define the genotype and endophenotype. Such research may contribute to the categorization and assessment of individuals with eating disorders.

Introduction

The aim of this review is to provide an update on recent findings from neuroimaging that pertain to eating disorders. The studies have been divided into four sections:

1 those that have examined the structure of the brain
2 those that have examined cerebral function by means of blood flow changes in resting conditions
3 those that have examined cerebral function by means of blood flow following salient cues, including food and body image, considering both satiated and hungry states
4 those that have examined neurotransmitter function.

It is essential to put neuroimaging results in eating disorders into context, but difficult to do so without some understanding of the central control of feeding, reward and emotional regulation, in order to consider neuroimaging findings in perspective. Therefore, a summary of this follows. The interested reader may wish to supplement this with further information; the work of Rolls (2005) offers an excellent overview.

Central control of feeding, reward and emotional regulation

The central control of food intake is summarized in Figure 7.1. There are two interdependent systems:

1 The *nutrostat* is a homeostatic system that links somatic sensors and metabolic signals with autonomic nervous activity and the regulation of food intake. The nutrostat system is a network within the central core of the brain, running from the brainstem to the forebrain.
2 The *hedonic/drive system* mediates the rewarding nature of food. It controls reward more generally and is also involved in motivation and emotional regulation. The hedonic/drive system lies in the next layer to the nutrostat, involving a network running from the orbitofrontal cortex, amygdala and striatum to the midbrain (O'Doherty *et al.* 2006).

The nutrostat sets the sensitivity of the hedonic/drive system to food. Thus, the reward value of food varies according to the level of metabolic depletion.

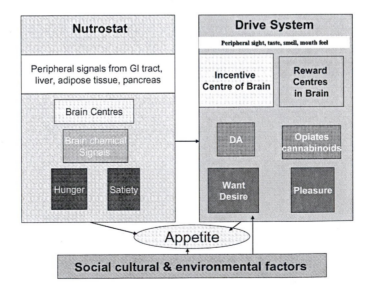

Figure 7.1   An illustration of the central control of appetite.

Literature review

Examining the structure of the brain

Pathological anomalies and eating disorder symptoms

Uher and Treasure (2005) summarized the literature describing structural anomalies in the brain associated with eating disorder syndromes. Brain lesions in the prefrontal, temporal and mesiotemporal regions and the hypothalamus, predominantly on the right-hand side, were found to be associated with pathological eating behaviors (Uher and Treasure 2005).

Brain structural findings in individuals with eating disorders

It is well documented that brain substance is reduced in individuals with eating disorders, particularly anorexia nervosa. However, a study of 40 people who had fully recovered from their eating disorder (i.e. were asymptomatic for over one year and had normal physiology) found that the brain volume was normal in size (Wagner *et al.* 2006). This suggests that the brain shrinkage is a reversible form of pseudo-atrophy, and is a probable consequence of the acute metabolic disruption. This may be due to starvation, or stress, or a combination of both.

The hippocampus is particularly vulnerable to shrinkage when cortisol levels are high. The hypothalamic–pituitary axis is deregulated in anorexia nervosa, and cortisol levels are increased. Therefore the finding that the hippocampus on both sides of the brain was particularly reduced in volume compared with the rest of the brain in individuals with anorexia nervosa was not unexpected (Connan *et al.* 2006). Interestingly, there was no detectable impairment of memory function. Thus loss of brain substance in eating disorders may not be associated with functional changes, or possibly other areas may compensate for any deficits.

Examining cerebral function in the resting state

Researchers have used positron emission tomography (PET) and single photon emission computed tomography (SPECT) to measure cerebral blood flow during resting conditions. As radiation is involved in this technology, it is unusual to have a matched control group in these studies. This means that the interpretation of results can be difficult.

Key and colleagues reported a reduction in basal blood flow in the anterior temporal and caudate regions in eight out of 11 of patients with anorexia nervosa (Key *et al.* 2006). This replicates the previous observations made by this group in adolescents with anorexia nervosa. Kojima and colleagues reported similar findings of reduced basal flow in the right parietal, occipital and insular cortex, and in the anterior cingulate cortex of patients with eating disorders compared with controls (Kojima *et al.* 2005).

Correlation of resting blood flow with clinical state

Some groups have attempted to correlate basal blood flow in individuals with eating disorders with aspects of their psychopathology or neuropsychological function. For example, Ferro and colleagues reported that performance on the classical Stroop Interference Task was correlated with activity in the superior frontal gyrus (four of the 16 patients with anorexia nervosa performed below one standard deviation from literature norms for this task) (Ferro *et al.* 2005). Goethals *et al.* (2006) reported that the level of body dissatisfaction in 67 patients with eating disorders was correlated with flow in the left ventromedial prefrontal cortex and right medial parietal areas. Furthermore, the subjective sense of ineffectiveness correlated with flow in the lateral ventral prefrontal cortex and left medial parietal areas (Goethals *et al.* 2006). Two longitudinal studies from Japan have found changes in cerebral blood flow after weight gain in patients with anorexia nervosa. Matsumoto and colleagues found increased blood flow in the anterior and posterior cingulate, the medial and dorsolateral prefrontal cortex and the precuneus (Matsumoto *et al.* 2006). Kojima and colleagues found increased blood flow in the right parietal area and decreased blood flow in the cerebellum and basal ganglia (Kojima *et al.* 2005).

Examining cerebral function following salient cues

There are several technical issues that need to be considered before interpreting the response of the brain to salient eating disorder cues. The centres involved in the hedonic response to food, such as the orbitofrontal cortex (OFC), may be subject to susceptibility artefacts, and this is poorly addressed in some functional magnetic resonance imaging (fMRI) studies. The baseline physiology, hunger, blood glucose level, etc., may vary between groups and act as significant confounding factors.

Several studies have examined the response to food in both the hungry and satiated state, in which the response to satiation typically follows the experimental paradigm in the hungry state. This fixed repetition of the experiment within a short time period is not controlled for. Furthermore, if meals are given these are often adjusted for body weight and therefore vary in size.

The instructions and the required response to the cues can have a profound effect on the results. Rolls and colleagues exemplified this by assigning visual labels to a standard olfactory cue, alternating between 'cheddar cheese' and 'body odour'. The anterior cingulate and OFC were activated more in response to the label 'cheddar cheese'. The difference in activation was linked to the subjective evaluation of pleasantness (de Araujo *et al.* 2005). All of these technical aspects mean that it can be difficult to obtain a coherent understanding of brain function.

Food stimuli

NORMAL SUBJECTS

STAGE OF DEVELOPMENT

Food stimuli in the fasting state in children and adolescents activate similar networks to those seen in adults. The amygdala (although this response habituates), orbitofrontal cortex, medial frontal cortex, cerebellum and fusiform cortex are all involved (Holsen *et al.* 2005).

REWARD SENSITIVITY

In response to high-palatability food, Beaver and colleagues found that the level of activation in the frontostriatal-amygdala network is correlated with the individual's self-reported reward sensitivity (Beaver *et al.* 2006). In subjects within the normal BMI range, Killgore found a negative relationship between BMI and activation in the reward areas of the brain in response to images of high-calorie food. This suggests that the rewarding properties of the food were more salient in individuals in the lower part of the normal BMI range (sensitivity to reward was not measured in this experiment) (Killgore and Yurgelun-Todd 2005).

COMPARISON BETWEEN THE HUNGRY AND NON-HUNGRY STATES

In theory both the nutrostat and the hedonic system may show differences in activation between the fasted and fed state. The response to food stimuli (images and taste) was compared following a 24-hour fast (when hunger and free fatty acid levels were increased, and insulin and leptin levels were decreased) and in the satiated state in 10 women and eight men (Uher *et al.* 2006). The visual food stimuli produced specific activation bilaterally in the fusiform and lingual gyri, and in the right angular gyrus and left anterior insula. The taste stimuli elicited activation in the dorsolateral prefrontal cortex. Visual but not taste food stimuli were perceived to be more pleasant in the fasted state. In the fasted state, activation in the left anterior insula and adjacent dorsolateral prefrontal cortex in response to taste stimuli was increased. There was a trend for the activation in the fusiform gyrus to be increased with the visual food stimuli in the fasted state. The interpretation of these findings is that hunger modulates the processing of food-related stimuli in the modality-specific sensory cortices. Interestingly, women showed greater responses to these food cues than men.

COMPARISON BETWEEN OBESE AND LEAN CONTROLS

Obese men showed less activation in the left dorsolateral prefrontal cortex in response to a meal than did normal men (Le *et al.* 2006). This is interesting, as earlier research with individuals with bulimia nervosa suggested that there was less activation to food cues in this area (Uher *et al.* 2004).

GENDER DIFFERENCES

Some studies suggest that there are gender differences in the response to food stimuli. For example, in men who were fed to satiety with chocolate, further chocolate tasting activated the reward centre of the brain, but this did not occur in women (Smeets *et al.* 2006). The gender difference in the response to food is of particular relevance to the development of eating disorders.

EATING-DISORDERED SUBJECTS

ANOREXIA NERVOSA

Santel and colleagues compared the response to images of high-calorie food in 13 people with anorexia nervosa with that of 10 controls (Santel *et al.* 2006). In individuals with anorexia nervosa there was bilateral activation in the occipital cortex and cerebellum in the satiated state, and in the right fusiform gyrus and occipital cortex in the hungry state. Occipital activation was greater in the satiated state than in the hungry state.

Compared with controls, individuals with AN showed less activation in the left inferior parietal region in the satiated state, and less activation in the occipital region in the hungry state. Activation in both of these regions was correlated with facets of psychopathology such as BMI, drive for thinness, and a sense of ineffectiveness. One interpretation of these findings is that images of high-calorie food were less salient in people with anorexia nervosa.

BINGE EATING

Geliebter and colleagues compared brain activation in response to food stimuli (visual images of binge and non-binge food) and auditory stimuli (food names) in 10 binge eaters (five obese and five normal-weight individuals) and 10 controls, three hours after eating a 650-kilocalorie meal (Geliebter *et al.* 2006). All of the groups showed activation of the occipital and temporal cortex in response to food stimuli. The obese binge-eating group showed greater activation in response to food stimuli in the frontal cortex (premotor area and inferior frontal gyrus), and in the occipital and temporal lobe (fusiform gyrus). This suggests that food stimuli had more salience in the obese binge-eating group.

Frank and colleagues examined activation in response to a glucose taste challenge in individuals who had recovered from a bulimic illness compared with normal controls (Frank *et al.* 2006). They reported that individuals with a history of bulimia showed less activation in the anterior cingulate and occipital cortex than the control group. The authors speculated that the decreased activation of limbic/reward systems might represent a decreased sensitivity to the reward of sweetness in this patient group.

Body image stimuli

Internalization of a thin ideal fosters body dissatisfaction, which is a key precipitating and perpetuating factor in eating disorders (Stice 2002). Several groups have examined brain activation in response to body image paradigms.

NORMAL SUBJECTS

Exposure to distorted self-images activates the limbic area and attention networks in normal female subjects (Kurosaki *et al.* 2006). There were gender differences in that the limbic system was not activated in normal male subjects. Other gender differences were found when derogatory words concerning body image were used. In females this activated the amygdala, whereas in males a wider network within the frontal lobe was activated (Shirao *et al.* 2005). These studies fit within the context of earlier investigations, and suggest that a neural network is involved in the general processing of body shapes (the lateral fusiform, parietal and dorsolateral prefrontal cortices), and a related "emotional" network (the anterior cingulate, insula and amygdala) is activated when the body-shape-related stimuli carry self-related or emotionally significant information. Women are particularly susceptible to activation of the emotional network in response to body image paradigms.

EATING-DISORDERED SUBJECTS

Simple line drawings of female bodies of different sizes (underweight, normal and overweight) were compared with line drawings of houses in 22 patients with eating disorders and 18 control subjects. Although the overweight and underweight female body shapes were subjectively rated as more aversive than the normal body shapes, the pattern of fMRI response to female body shapes was similar across different categories of stimuli (underweight, normal and overweight) and across groups of participating women (with or without an eating disorder). Activation was distributed in a network that included the lateral fusiform gyrus, the lateral prefrontal cortex (PFC) and the right parietal cortex (Uher *et al.* 2005a). The patients with eating disorders showed a generally weaker response to body shapes in the occipitotemporal and parietal cortices than did the healthy women.

With regard to subjective reaction, a large range was reported in the eating-disordered group. Aversion ratings to the body images were positively associated with activity in the apical medial prefrontal cortex, and negatively associated with the activity in the left lateral fusiform gyrus. An index of body image disturbance (relative aversion to normal versus thin bodies) correlated positively with a cluster of activity in the inferior medial temporal lobe, including the medial aspect of the amygdala. The latter correlation was largely due to three cases with severe body image disturbance and high reactivity to body shapes in this region. Thus these images activated the 'emotional' system in some women with eating disorders.

Examining neurotransmitter function

Brain imaging studies using neurotransmitter ligands offer the potential to understand the chemistry of brain function. Dopamine, opiates and serotonin (5HT) are of particular interest because of their role in the nutrostat and hedonic systems that control eating.

Dopamine

The dopamine system is thought to play a key role in the hedonic system – that is, the drive to seek rewards. There is evidence that the dopamine system is disrupted in individuals with anorexia nervosa. Frank and colleagues found that, after recovery from anorexia nervosa (normal weight regained), raclopride binding is increased in the anterior striatum (Frank *et al.* 2005). This indicates increased availability of dopamine D2 receptors, which suggests that basal tonic dopamine release is reduced. This has parallels with the findings of Wang and colleagues that BMI at the obese end of the spectrum correlated negatively with striatal D2 receptors (Wang *et al.* 2001). Thus obese individuals have fewer 'empty' D2 receptors, indicating higher basal tonic dopamine release. Lower tonic dopamine release in the striatum in individuals with anorexia nervosa may alter the setting of reward, reducing the drive to eat.

An increase in empty dopamine D2 receptors is seen in other conditions, such as children born preterm and with poor neonatal blood flow (Lou *et al.* 2004). This is of interest, given the known association of adverse perinatal factors with the later development of eating disorders (Favaro *et al.* 2006).

Serotonin

The serotonin system is thought to be part of the punishment system that counteracts the reward system. Kaye's model of anorexia nervosa suggests that increased 5HT activity is a vulnerability factor for the development of anorexia nervosa. The theory postulates that 5HT homeostasis is disrupted by dieting. Food restriction reduces tryptophan intake, and the production of 5HT is reduced. The consequent reduction in central 5HT release reduces anxiety and produces a sense of well-being which is reinforcing (Kaye *et al.* 2001). There is some evidence from neurochemical imaging studies that supports this hypothesis.

Individuals with anorexia nervosa have anomalies in the serotonin system both in the acute state and after recovery.

Anorexia nervosa

Bailer and colleagues found an increase in 5HT1A binding throughout many brain regions in the acute phase of anorexia nervosa, although the number of

5HT2A receptors did not differ from that in the control population (Bailer *et al.* 2007).

Anorexia nervosa binge–purge subtype

Reduced 5HT2A binding in the parietal area was found in individuals in the acute phase of the binge–purge subtype of anorexia nervosa in a SPECT study (Goethals *et al.* 2005). The receptor levels correlated with the trait of reward dependence. In a separate study, subjects who had recovered from the binge–purge subtype of AN also showed reduced 5HT2A binding in the subgenual cingulate region (Bailer *et al.* 2004).

Furthermore, similar subjects (post-recovery binge–purge subtype) showed a widespread increase in 5HT1A binding (Bailer *et al.* 2005). The level of binding to receptors in the medial temporal and subgenual cingulate region correlated with harm avoidance. The 5HT1A receptors are commonly autoreceptors on the cell body of 5HT neurons, and reduce synaptic 5HT release.

Opiates

The opiate system is thought to mediate the consummatory pleasure aspect of reward. Preliminary evidence suggests that this system is deregulated in people with eating disorders. Subjects with bulimia nervosa ($n = 8$) showed a 17% decrease in ì-opiate receptors (carefentanil) in the left insular cortex. This correlated with their recent fasting behavior (Bencherif *et al.* 2005). This interesting preliminary finding suggests that further research on the reward mechanisms in eating disorders is needed.

Clinical implications

It is uncertain whether any of these findings can be translated into clinical treatment at the present time. In a pilot study, Uher and colleagues administered blindly to women who reported high levels of food craving either real or sham repetitive transcranial magnetic stimulation (TMS) to an area over the right dorsolateral cortex (an area that shows decreased activation in individuals with bulimia nervosa) (Uher *et al.* 2005b). Craving for food gradually increased over the course of the experiment in those who were administered the sham TMS. However, the women who were administered the real TMS showed no change in the level of craving over the course of the experiment. Nevertheless, the actual amount of snack food eaten showed no significant difference between the two groups. It is therefore uncertain whether such a decrease in craving might be of value to people with clinical eating disorders.

The specificity of the balance of receptor profiles within specific eating disorder subgroups (e.g. the 5HT system and binge–purge anorexia nervosa) suggests that a future goal will be to tailor pharmacological treatment to the individual.

Conclusion

It is difficult to draw firm conclusions from the neuroimaging research published in 2005 and 2006. This is still very much 'work in progress', and it is not easy to draw out consistent themes. However, the neurochemical dissection of brain function is starting to form a coherent story. Thus there appears to be an imbalance between dopamine and serotonin pathways, which may relate to differential sensitivity of the reward and punishment mechanism across the different forms of eating disorders. Expanding this line of research into other aspects of the reward pathway, such as opiate and cannabinoid mechanisms, may complete the picture. This may explain the link to leanness for anorexia nervosa (Hebebrand and Remschmidt 1995) and to obesity for the binge-eating disorders.

The plasticity of the brain is an area of active research. This may explain how and why recovery from eating disorder symptoms becomes more difficult the longer an eating disorders persists. The gross loss in brain substance (particularly in the hippocampus) caused by malnutrition resolves with recovery. However, it is possible that appetite and reward systems may become permanently disrupted by a prolonged period of starvation. Research involving animal models suggest that this is an important possibility (Hagan *et al.* 2003; Boggiano *et al.* 2005; Avena *et al.* 2006; Corwin 2006). It will be of interest to examine changes in brain function following treatment.

More research is needed to elucidate fully the perceptual, emotional and cognitive underpinnings of eating disorders. One strategy will be to devise scanning experiments which define the genotype and endophenotype. This has been a successful approach in other branches of psychiatry. There are interesting leads, such as the links between developmental adversity, emotional processing and the 5HT genotype and endophenotype in the bulimic disorders (Steiger and Bruce 2007), and the links between information processing and OCPD personality traits in anorexia nervosa (Treasure 2007).

References

(References included from the targeted review years are preceded by one asterisk. References preceded by three asterisks are of particular significance. The significance is explained by a short commentary following the complete reference.)

*Avena NM, Rada P, Moise N and Hoebel BG (2006) Sucrose sham feeding on a binge schedule releases accumbens dopamine repeatedly and eliminates the acetylcholine satiety response. *Neuroscience*, **139:** 813–20.

*Bailer UF, Price JC, Meltzer CC, Mathis CA, Frank GK, Weissfeld L *et al.* (2004) Altered 5-HT(2A) receptor binding after recovery from bulimia-type anorexia nervosa: relationships to harm avoidance and drive for thinness. *Neuropsychopharmacology*, **29:** 1143–55.

*Bailer UF, Frank GK, Henry SE, Price JC, Meltzer CC, Weissfeld L *et al.* (2005) Altered brain serotonin 5-HT1A receptor binding after recovery from anorexia nervosa measured by positron emission tomography and [carbonyl11C]WAY-100635. *Archives of General Psychiatry*, **62**: 1032–41.

*Bailer UF, Frank GK, Henry SE, Price JC, Meltzer CC, Mathis CA *et al.* (2007) Exaggerated 5-HT1A but normal 5-HT2A receptor activity in individuals ill with anorexia nervosa. *Biological Psychiatry*, **61**: 1090–99.

*Beaver JD, Lawrence AD, van Ditzhuijzen J, Davis MH, Woods A and Calder AJ (2006) Individual differences in reward drive predict neural responses to images of food. *Journal of Neuroscience*, **26**: 5160–66.

***Bencherif B, Guarda AS, Colantuoni C, Ravert HT, Dannals RF and Frost JJ (2005) Regional mu-opioid receptor binding in insular cortex is decreased in bulimia nervosa and correlates inversely with fasting behavior. *Journal of Nuclear Medicine*, **46**: 1349–51. **This interesting preliminary study of potential changes within the opiate system in eating disorders has pertinent findings that link in with theories of reward mechanisms. The correlation with recent fasting behavior is particularly notable. This paper leads the way for future studies to add further clarification to the neurochemical basis of eating disorders within the context of reward systems.**

*Boggiano MM, Chandler PC, Viana JB, Oswald KD, Maldonado CR and Wauford PK (2005) Combined dieting and stress evoke exaggerated responses to opioids in binge-eating rats. *Behavioral Neuroscience*, **119**: 1207–14.

*Connan F, Murphy F, Connor SE, Rich P, Murphy T, Bara-Carill N *et al.* (2006) Hippocampal volume and cognitive function in anorexia nervosa. *Psychiatry Research*, **146**: 117–25.

*Corwin RL (2006) Bingeing rats: a model of intermittent excessive behavior? *Appetite*, **46**: 11–15.

*de Araujo IE, Rolls ET, Velazco MI, Margot C and Cayeux I (2005) Cognitive modulation of olfactory processing. *Neuron*, **46**: 671–9.

*Favaro A, Tenconi E and Santonastaso P (2006) Perinatal factors and the risk of developing anorexia nervosa and bulimia nervosa. *Archives of General Psychiatry*, **63**: 82–8.

*Ferro AM, Brugnolo A, De Leo C, Dessi B, Girtler N, Morbelli S *et al.* (2005) Stroop interference task and single-photon emission tomography in anorexia: a preliminary report. *International Journal of Eating Disorders*, **38**: 323–9.

***Frank GK, Bailer UF, Henry SE, Drevets W, Meltzer CC, Price JC *et al.* (2005) Increased dopamine D2/D3 receptor binding after recovery from anorexia nervosa measured by positron emission tomography and [11c]raclopride. *Biological Psychiatry*, **58**: 908–12. **This paper is part of a series of investigations which have examined the neurochemistry of individuals with eating disorders in a normal physiological state after recovery. This study suggests that anomalies of the dopamine system are present in individuals with anorexia nervosa. It would be interesting to ascertain whether this is a vulnerability trait or a "scar" effect.**

*Frank GK, Wagner A, Achenbach S, McConaha C, Skovira K, Aizenstein H *et al.* (2006) Altered brain activity in women recovered from bulimic-type eating disorders after a glucose challenge: a pilot study. *International Journal of Eating Disorders*, **39**: 76–9.

*Geliebter A, Ladell T, Logan M, Schweider T, Sharafi M and Hirsch J (2006) Responsivity to food stimuli in obese and lean binge eaters using functional MRI. *Appetite*, **46**: 31–5.

*Goethals I, Vervaet M, Audenaert K, Jacobs F, Ham H, Van de Wiele C *et al.* (2007) Differences of cortical 5-HT(2A) receptor binding index with SPECT in subtypes of anorexia nervosa: relationship with personality traits? *Journal of Psychiatric Research*, **41**: 455–8.

*Goethals I, Vervaet M, Audenaert K, Jacobs F, Ham H and van Heeringen C (2006) Does regional brain perfusion correlate with eating disorder symptoms in anorexia and bulimia nervosa patients? *Journal of Psychiatric Research*, 41(12): 1005–11.

*Hagan MM, Chandler PC, Wauford PK, Rybak RJ and Oswald KD (2003) The role of palatable food and hunger as trigger factors in an animal model of stress-induced binge eating. *International Journal of Eating Disorders*, **34**: 183–97.

*Hebebrand J and Remschmidt H (1995) Anorexia nervosa viewed as an extreme weight condition: genetic implications. *Human Genetics*, **95**: 1–11.

*Holsen LM, Zarcone JR, Thompson TI, Brooks WM, Anderson MF, Ahluwalia JS *et al.* (2005) Neural mechanisms underlying food motivation in children and adolescents. *Neuroimage*, **27**: 669–76.

*Kaye W, Gendall K and Strober M (2001) Nutrition, serotonin and behavior in anorexia and bulimia nervosa. *Nestlé Nutrition Workshop Series. Clinical and Performance Programme*, **5**: 153–65.

*Key A, O'Brien A, Gordon I, Christie D and Lask B (2006) Assessment of neurobiology in adults with anorexia nervosa. *European Eating Disorder Review*, **14**: 308–14.

*Killgore WD and Yurgelun-Todd DA (2005) Body mass predicts orbitofrontal activity during visual presentations of high-calorie foods. *Neuroreport*, **16**: 859–63.

*Kojima S, Nagai N, Nakabeppu Y, Muranaga T, Deguchi D, Nakajo M *et al.* (2005) Comparison of regional cerebral blood flow in patients with anorexia nervosa before and after weight gain. *Psychiatry Research*, **140**: 251–8.

*Kurosaki M, Shirao N, Yamashita H, Okamoto Y and Yamawaki S (2006) Distorted images of one's own body activate the prefrontal cortex and limbic/paralimbic system in young women: a functional magnetic resonance imaging study. *Biological Psychiatry*, **59**: 380–86.

*Le DS, Pannacciulli N, Chen K, Del Parigi A, Salbe AD, Reiman EM *et al.* (2006) Less activation of the left dorsolateral prefrontal cortex in response to a meal: a feature of obesity. *American Journal of Clinical Nutrition*, **84**: 725–31.

*Lou HC, Rosa P, Pryds O, Karrebaek H, Lunding J, Cumming P *et al.* (2004) ADHD: increased dopamine receptor availability linked to attention deficit and low neonatal cerebral blood flow. *Developmental Medicine and Child Neurology*, **46**: 179–83.

*Matsumoto R, Kitabayashi Y, Narumoto J, Wada Y, Okamoto A, Ushijima Y *et al.* (2006) Regional cerebral blood flow changes associated with interoceptive awareness in the recovery process of anorexia nervosa. *Progress in Neuro-Psychopharmacology and Biological Psychiatry*, **30**: 1265–70.

***O'Doherty JP, Buchanan TW, Seymour B and Dolan RJ (2006) Predictive neural coding of reward preference involves dissociable responses in human ventral midbrain and ventral striatum. *Neuron*, **49**: 157–66.
   This paper is one of a series by the same authors that are interrogating human reward mechanisms.

*Rolls ET (2005) Taste, olfactory and food texture processing in the brain, and the control of food intake. *Physiology and Behavior*, **85**: 45–56.

***Santel S, Baving L, Krauel K, Munte TF and Rotte M (2006) Hunger and satiety in anorexia nervosa: fMRI during cognitive processing of food pictures. *Brain Research*, **1114**: 138–48.
   This robust study postulates potential mechanisms of altered cognitive processing of visual food stimuli in anorexia nervosa.

*Shirao N, Okamoto Y, Mantani T, Okamoto Y and Yamawaki S (2005) Gender differences in brain activity generated by unpleasant word stimuli concerning body image: an fMRI study. *British Journal of Psychiatry*, **186**: 48–53.

*Smeets PA, de Graaf C, Stafleu A, van Osch MJ, Nievelstein RA and van der Grond J (2006) Effect of satiety on brain activation during chocolate tasting in men and women. *American Journal of Clinical Nutrition*, **83**: 1297–305.

*Steiger H and Bruce K (2007) Phenotypes, endophenotypes and genotypes in bulimia-spectrum eating disorders. *Canadian Journal of Psychiatry*, **52**: 220–27.

*Stice E (2002) Risk and maintenance factors for eating pathology: a meta-analytic review. *Psychology Bulletin*, **128**: 825–48.

*Treasure J (2007) Getting beneath the phenotype of anorexia nervosa: the search for viable endophenotypes and genotypes. *Canadian Journal of Psychiatry*, **52**: 212–19.

*Uher R and Treasure J (2005) Brain lesions and eating disorders. *Journal of Neurology, Neurosurgery and Psychiatry*, **76**: 852–7.

*Uher R, Murphy T, Brammer MJ, Dalgleish T, Phillips ML, Ng VW *et al.* (2004) Medial prefrontal cortex activity associated with symptom provocation in eating disorders. *American Journal of Psychiatry*, **161**: 1238–46.

*Uher R, Murphy T, Friederich HC, Dalgleish T, Brammer MJ, Giampietro V *et al.* (2005a) Functional neuroanatomy of body shape perception in healthy and eating-disordered women. *Biological Psychiatry*, **58**: 990–97.

*Uher R, Yoganathan D, Mogg A, Eranti SV, Treasure J, Campbell IC *et al.* (2005b) Effect of left prefrontal repetitive transcranial magnetic stimulation on food craving. *Biological Psychiatry*, **58**: 840–42.

*Uher R, Treasure J, Heining M, Brammer MJ and Campbell IC (2006) Cerebral processing of food-related stimuli: effects of fasting and gender. *Behavioural Brain Research*, **169**: 111–19.

*Wagner A, Greer P, Bailer UF, Frank GK, Henry SE, Putnam K *et al.* (2006) Normal brain tissue volumes after long-term recovery in anorexia and bulimia nervosa. *Biological Psychiatry*, **59**: 291–3.

*Wang GJ, Volkow ND, Logan J, Pappas NR, Wong CT, Zhu W *et al.* (2001) Brain dopamine and obesity. *Lancet*, **357**: 354–7.

8

Eating disorders in children and adolescents

Maria Øverås, Eirin Winje and Bryan Lask

Abstract

Objectives of review. The aim of this chapter is to review papers published in 2005 and 2006 specifically relating to children and adolescents with eating disorders, in order to identify significant new findings and explore future research requirements.

Summary of recent findings. There is increasing evidence that anorexia nervosa may commonly have a neurodevelopmental substrate. Comorbidity and potentially serious physical complications are common, but receive insufficient attention. There has been an increasing emphasis on seeing parents as a resource and on enhancing their coping and management skills. Dependence upon weight or BMI and on self-report of menstruation to determine changes in management or to define outcome has no scientific basis. There is limited evidence for the effectiveness of specific treatments, and the clinically sound enthusiasm for family-based treatments lacks empirical support.

Future directions. There is a need to understand better the possible role of a neurobiological substrate, to use the same outcome criteria across studies, and for better designed studies of both specific and combined therapies.

Introduction

The number of publications relating to child and adolescent eating disorders continues to increase. In this review of the literature published in 2005 and 2006, we focus on assessment, incidence and prevalence, physical, psychological and family correlates, and treatment and outcome, and reflect the strong emphasis on physical complications and parent and family issues. We end with a summary of the findings, consider the clinical implications and make some recommendations about future research directions.

Assessment

The assessment of eating disorder psychopathology in children and adolescents is more complex than that of adults, not least because reports come from multiple sources. Consequently, the need to establish effective, reliable and valid instruments for this age group has received much attention. Watkins *et al.* (2005), in their study of the Eating Disorder Examination (EDE) adapted for children (ChEDE), showed that this instrument has a high degree of internal consistency, discriminant validity and inter-rater reliability. Binford *et al.* (2005) found the adult version of the EDE and the questionnaire form (EDE-Q) in adolescents to be only moderately correlated. To better capture the anorexia nervosa (AN) symptomatology, Couturier and Lock (2006a) added eight items to the EDE, which increased its internal validity. However, it seems more appropriate to use the ChEDE or to include a parent component (Binford *et al.* 2005; Courturier and Lock 2006a).

Information provided by or about the parents can prove invaluable. Lask *et al.* (2005a) have shown that a single consultation (almost always parent-instigated) with the family physician about eating, weight or shape concerns is a strong predictor of the subsequent emergence of AN within 12 months. A core component of family therapy is to enhance parental skills in their management of the illness. The Parents Versus Anorexia Scale (PVA) was developed as a means of evaluating this. Rhodes *et al.* (2005) have provided support for its validity by showing a significant difference between the scores of parents whose children responded well to treatment compared with the scores of parents on a waiting list.

Incidence and prevalence

Estimating the incidence/prevalence of eating disorders is always challenging, and all the more so in children and adolescents who generally tend to conceal their illness. Rodriguez-Cano *et al.* (2005) found a prevalence of 3.7% of adolescents in Spain, but the rate of false negatives in the control group was 2.6%, suggesting that this was an underestimation of the prevalence.

A further confounding factor is the possibility that the presentation of eating disorders may vary between different cultural/ethnic groups. For example, Tareen *et al.* (2005) found that South Asian adolescents with AN who were living in the UK were significantly less likely than adolescents in the white population to present with fat phobia or to express a preoccupation with food and weight. They were also less likely to over-exercise in order to control their weight. In contrast, Lee *et al.* (2005) reported that the clinical picture of patients living in Singapore resembles that in Western countries. In a Latina subsample of US adolescents, Granillo *et al.* (2005) found that the Latina subgroup was less likely than the rest of the sample to have a BMI of 17 or less and a greater level of dietary restraint. There was no difference with regard to bulimic behavior between the two groups. Higher socioeconomic status of the parents was a risk factor for eating disorders in the Latina subgroup.

Physical correlates

Eating disorders in childhood and adolescence are associated with a very wide range of physical problems, with every body system at risk. Reduced bone density (osteopenia or osteoporosis) is one of the most commonly reported complications, and three recent studies provide further evidence for this (Bass *et al.* 2005; Konstantynowicz *et al.* 2005; Compston *et al.* 2006). In the first of these studies it was also noted that the reduction in bone density was much higher in those patients who were depressed. With weight restoration, both linear growth (Compston *et al.* 2006) and increase in bone density (Bass *et al.* 2005) were reported. A key factor in restoring bone density is the resumption of menses. However, self-reports concerning menstruation may not always be accurate. Swenne *et al.* (2005) found a divergence in self-reported menstrual status between interviews. Furthermore, 25% of teenage girls who were on the contraceptive pill were reported as menstruating. Abraham *et al.* (2005) have also questioned the usefulness of amenorrhea as a diagnostic and outcome criterion, on the basis that it cannot be assessed for many of the younger age groups in females, and not at all in males.

AN is associated with abnormalities in vital organs such as the heart and brain. Both Olivares *et al.* (2005) and Ulger *et al.* (2006) reported significant structural and functional cardiac anomalies, but these were reversible with adequate re-feeding.

Lask *et al.* (2005b) have noted that approximately 70% of children and adolescents with AN have a significant reduction in blood flow (indicating hypometabolism) in the limbic system, and neurocognitive deficits, neither of which seem to be reversible with nutritional restoration. They conclude that these findings reflect a primary abnormality in the cortico-striatal system, which may be a necessary substrate for some cases of early-onset AN.

Favaro *et al.* (2006) have also proposed a neurodevelopmental etiology in AN, noting a high rate of various obstetric complications which proved to be significant and independent risk factors for its emergence. The risk increased with the total number of obstetric complications, and the number of complications was inversely correlated with the age of onset of AN. Obstetric complications were also significantly associated with bulimia nervosa (BN).

Finally, in relation to the brain, Rohrer *et al.* (2006) have offered yet another report of failure to diagnose a tumor because of the clinician's failure to think 'outside the box'. The moral of the tale is that not every case of food avoidance and weight loss in adolescence is due to an eating disorder, and that all clinicians should be mindful of the possibility of covert brain disease.

In contrast, the skin often reveals features of hidden eating disorders, such as peripheral circulatory insufficiency, hypercarotenemia, parotid gland enlargement and Russell's sign, or evidence of trauma to the dorsum of the hand caused by inducing vomiting with the hand (Strumia 2005). The teeth may also reveal signs of covert eating disorders, specifically dental erosion (Imfeld and Imfeld 2005). These authors argue that the main goals of dental care are to preserve the remaining teeth and to prevent further erosion, and that dental restorative therapy should be part of comprehensive treatment.

Psychological correlates

Just as adolescents and adults with eating disorders may differ, so may children and adolescents. Peebles *et al.* (2006) found important diagnostic and gender differences, with children more likely to be male, to present with an 'atypical' eating disorder, to engage in less binge-eating and purging, and to have a lower percentage ideal body weight, having lost weight more rapidly. There was less BN in the younger group, but the prevalence of AN and comorbidity were the same in the two age groups.

The commonest comorbidities in patients with eating disorders are mood and anxiety disorders (e.g. Blinder *et al.* 2006), but such studies have tended to focus on adults, or have failed to distinguish between adolescents and adults (McDermott *et al.* 2006). Serpell *et al.* (2006) and McDermott *et al.* (2006) have looked specifically at the prevalence of comorbid psychopathology in adolescents with eating disorders. Serpell *et al.* (2006) found that about half of their population of adolescents with AN had clinically significant symptoms of obsessive-compulsive disorder (OCD), but only a small percentage of the young patients with AN had obsessive-compulsive personality traits. These authors also pointed out that it is inappropriate to seek or make a diagnosis of personality disorder in the younger population, as personality is not yet fully developed, and some behaviors may be more a reflection of age than of personality disorder.

McDermott *et al.* (2006) found the same rate of depression and anxiety in adolescents with eating disorders as in a control group of young patients with a primary diagnosis of mood or anxiety disorder. Furthermore, patients with AN scored significantly lower on both externalizing and general psychopathology scores compared with patients with other eating disorders and a healthy control group. In line with findings in adults, these studies indicate high rates of comorbid psychopathology in adolescents with eating disorders.

Another question is how the comorbid disorders link to different aspects of the eating disorders. Serpell *et al.* (2006) found that high levels of comorbid psychopathology in patients with AN, but not in those with other eating disorders, predicted more severe eating disorder symptoms and longer duration of illness prior to the assessment. Ruuska *et al.* (2005) found a strong correlation between higher levels of psychological distress, measured by Symptom check list (SCL-90) and body dissatisfaction.

With regard to body image disturbance, Ruuska *et al.* (2005) found that adolescents with BN experienced more negative attitudes towards their own body than patients with AN, and Ravaldi *et al.* (2006) found a higher degree of body dissatisfaction in young ballet dancers than in a control group of non-dancers.

Several studies have also looked at gender differences in body image. For example, Eisenberg *et al.* (2006) found that on average adolescent boys had a more positive body image than adolescent girls. However, when Gila *et al.* (2005) compared young boys diagnosed with AN with a healthy group of boys, they found that the index group had significantly greater body dissatisfaction and body image disturbance. Furthermore, Eisenberg *et al.* (2006) showed that the body dissatisfaction of both girls and boys had increased after five years.

There has recently been growing interest in the field of neuropsychology and eating disorders. The findings seem to indicate that AN is associated with some kind of neuropsychological deficit (Duchesne *et al.* 2004), although the exact nature of these deficits and how they relate to the development and main- tainance of eating disorders is unclear. Also, since children and adolescents are still in a developmental stage, results from adult studies cannot automatically be generalized to the younger population. It is therefore important that separate studies are conducted with children and adolescents.

Using a range of computerized neuropsychological tests, Fowler *et al.* (2005) found significant deficits in spatial recognition memory, planning, and rapid visual information processing, unrelated to BMI, in adolescents with AN but not in healthy controls. The authors suggest that a neuropsychological deficit is not a general problem in AN, but may be a contributing factor for a subgroup of patients.

Pieters *et al.* (2005) followed up a group of young patients with AN who at low weight had shown faster motor speed compared with healthy controls, and found that the differences persisted after weight restoration. At both time points the patients with AN made significantly more errors than the control group, which could indicate a trade-off between speed and accuracy.

Family correlates

Much has been written in the past about the relationship between family functioning and eating disorders. Five recent studies shed some light on these possible associations. May *et al.* (2006) reported that increases in the weight concerns of girls, most commonly occurring between the ages of 11 and 16 years, were associated with increasing conflict with either parent and decreasing maternal intimacy and knowledge. In contrast, decreases in the weight concerns of boys, usually from the age of about 11 years, were associated with decreasing conflict with fathers.

Perkins *et al.* (2005) explored the reasons for adolescents with BN preferring not to include their parents in treatment. They found that patients who did not involve their parents in treatment tended to be older, had more chronic symptoms, exhibited more comorbid and impulsive behaviors, and perceived their mothers as having a more blaming and negative attitude towards the illness. They concluded that public awareness about BN needs to be raised, focusing on reducing the stigma and negative attitudes linked to the illness.

With regard to the previously very strongly expressed view that there is a specific and pathological pattern of family relationships associated with ado- lescent AN, Cook-Darzens *et al.* (2005), using a self-report measure that was completed by all family members, showed no evidence for such specificity and few differences compared with control families. There were some specific areas of distress and dissatisfaction which indicate that family therapists should adopt a more flexible view of family functioning, adapting therapeutic interventions to each family's individual style and level of functioning, and in particular focusing on all family members as a resource, not as a focus of pathology.

Davis *et al.* (2005) explored the association between the activity levels of adolescent girls with AN and their parents, compared with a control group of healthy girls and their parents. The patients with AN were on average more active than the controls. However, the activity level of adolescents and their parents was found to be related in both groups. In other words, if the parents were very active it was likely that their daughters would also be very active.

The subtleties and complexities noted from parental accounts of their coping strategies in the face of an eating disorder cannot be captured or categorized using conventional quantitative constructions of coping styles (Honey and Halse 2006). They call for the design of measures that accurately reflect parents' coping efforts. In a timely manner, Whitney *et al.* (2005) reported a qualitative study of the experience of caring for someone with AN. They found that carers experienced high levels of self-blame and helplessness, that mothers exhibited an intense emotional response and that fathers exhibited a more cognitive and detached response. They concluded that training parents in skills to manage the illness may improve outcome by reducing interpersonal maintaining factors.

Physical treatments

There are relatively few reports of physical treatments. Roots *et al.* (2006) studied the use of target weights during the inpatient treatment of adolescents with AN, and reported that there was considerable variation in how target weights are calculated, expected rates of weight gain, and the link between length of stay and attainment of targets. They concluded that there is little outcome evidence on which decisions can be based concerning these variables.

Two papers focused on the use of psychotropic medication. Holtkamp *et al.* (2005a) found in a retrospective study of adolescents with AN that selective serotonin reuptake inhibitors (SSRIs) had no appreciable effect on eating disorder psychopathology or on depressive or obsessive-compulsive comorbidity. They concluded that clinicians should be wary of using these drugs until there is more evidence for their efficacy. Reporting on an open trial of olanzapine, used as a supplement to psychotherapy, Dennis *et al.* (2006) noted decreased anxiety about eating, improved sleep, and decreased rumination about food and body concerns.

Finally, Golden *et al.* (2005) have reported a randomized, double-blind, placebo-controlled trial of alendroate (a bisphosphonate) for the treatment of osteopenia in AN. At follow-up, body weight was the most important determinant of bone mineral density, and there were no significant differences between those patients who received alendroate and individuals who received placebo. The authors concluded that alendroate should be confined to controlled clinical trials. In a critique of this study, Ott (2005) expressed concern about the trial, stating that bisphosphonates should not be used in females of child-bearing age, because of their potential to harm any subsequent fetus. In addition, such drugs can cause avascular osteonecrosis of the jaw (Landis *et al.*

2006). It is clear that their use in this age group, even in clinical trials, is strongly contraindicated.

Psychological treatments

Eating disorders have a poor prognosis, and more evidence-based knowledge of effective treatments is clearly needed, especially for the treatment of children and adolescents (Le Grange and Schmidt 2005). Lock (2005) has adapted a cognitive–behavioral therapy (CBT) manual, originally developed for treatment of adults with BN, for a younger population. Preliminary results suggest that this might be an appropriate and efficient way of treating children and adolescents with BN (Lock 2005; Schapman-Williams *et al.* 2006).

Offord *et al.* (2006) have interviewed young patients with AN after discharge from an inpatient unit. The patients found returning home difficult for a number of reasons, including the relative isolation from the outside world during hospitalization, and the differences between the hospital and the home environment with regard to structure, support and responsibility. The hospital structure and rules were seen as positive when staff offered an adequate rationale for them. However, patients highlighted the importance of staff gradually returning responsibility to them before discharge. In treatment, many patients reported feeling that staff based their approach too much on generalized assumptions about how a patient with AN thinks and behaves, rather than on the individual strengths and difficulties of each patient. Furthermore, patients gave more positive reports about treatment programs in which weight, shape and eating were not the sole focus, and where underlying problems such as low self-esteem or depressive thoughts were addressed. In general, a collaborative approach was seen as more helpful than a controlling one. Finally, although contact with other patients at the unit sometimes resulted in the learning of new unhealthy behaviors, most patients experienced the contact with other patients as an important source of support and motivation.

The majority of reported treatment has been family based. A recurrent theme has been the importance of actively including the parents in the treatment program. Most authors put a particular emphasis on enhancing family strengths (e.g. Eisler 2005; Honig 2005), rather than focusing on pathology. Many argue for the value of managing AN in the naturalistic context of home life rather than the clinical setting of an inpatient ward (e.g. Fleminger 2005; Honig 2005). Multi-family therapy is becoming increasingly popular, with important components including peer-group support, sharing of ideas and pooling of experience (e.g. Eisler 2005; Honig 2005; Scholz *et al.* 2005).

The majority of recently published papers on family-based treatments deal with outcome. Several authors (e.g. Fairburn 2005; Le Grange and Lock 2005) have drawn attention to the serious methodological inadequacies of most studies. Fairburn (2005) states that there is no convincing evidence for family-based treatments being a particularly effective therapy for adolescents with eating disorders, that all the studies to date have been too methodologically flawed to allow useful conclusions to be drawn, and that it is not clear from these studies that the effects which have been shown are due to family involvement. Lock and Le Grange (2005) agree that most studies have serious methodological problems, such as small sample size, samples that include only mild or moderate illness, or a lack of control groups. In addition, many studies use over-generous 'good' outcome criteria (e.g. 85% or more of ideal body weight), or rely upon self-report of menstrual status. Bergh *et al.* (2006) have summarized the situation by stating that the information currently available suggests that "family therapy may only be of some help for very mildly affected individuals, if it has any long-term effect at all".

The most recently published papers have attempted, with varying degrees of success, to address some but not all of these methodological inadequacies. Le Grange *et al.* (2005), among others, have argued for the importance of clinical trials being based upon manualized therapies. They reported the outcome of a case series of 45 mildly to moderately ill patients with AN, aged 9–18 years (mean age 14.5 years), who received an average of 17 sessions of manualized family therapy. However, only 56% had a good outcome, leaving almost half with an intermediate or poor outcome.

Lock *et al.* (2005, 2006a) have reported on a comparison of manualized short-term (10 sessions in six months) and long-term (20 sessions in 12 months) family therapy. Of 141 adolescents with mild to moderate AN who were eligible to participate, 86 individuals were recruited and randomized (44 to short-term and 42 to long-term therapy). At a mean follow-up of four years, nine individuals had discontinued the treatment and a further eight were not traced. Thus, follow-up information was available for 69 of the original 155 eligible patients (45%). Despite the low percentage, this represents a considerably higher number of patients than has been reported in other published studies. No differences were found between the two treatment modalities, and most patients did well, with 89% being above 90% of ideal body weight, and 74% of those who completed the EDE scoring within the normal range.

In the same sample, Lock *et al.* (2006b) reported on specific predictors of drop-out and remission. Higher rates of drop-out from family therapy (in a treatment trial) were associated with comorbid psychiatric disorder and longer treatment. Lower rates of remission were associated with comorbid psychiatric disorder, older age and problematic family behaviors. Higher rates of remission were associated with a reduction of child behavioral symptoms during treatment, a decline in problematic family behaviors, and early weight gain.

With regard to patient satisfaction, the findings are more encouraging. In one such study Paulson-Karlsson *et al.* (2006) found at an 18-month follow-up of family-based treatment, including individual, parent and family sessions, that 41 parents (83%) and 30 patients (73%) expressed satisfaction with the treatment. High levels of parent satisfaction have been reported for a parent psycho-education group in the treatment of adolescents with eating disorders (Hagenah and Vloet 2005), and for a group parent-training program (Zucker *et al.* 2006).

Outcome

It is remarkably difficult to compare outcomes between centres and between populations. Couturier and Lock (2006b, 2006c) have shown that there is enormous variation in the criteria used to define remission and recovery. They analysed a data set of 86 adolescents according to seven different criteria for remission. The definitions differed on parameters such as BMI, psychopathology, compensatory behaviors and menstrual status and how many of these were included. The different remission criteria gave a range of 3–96%, and the different recovery criteria gave a range of 57–94%, demonstrating the need for standardized definitions to be used in all outcome studies. This view renders the literature difficult to interpret.

This is illustrated by five follow-up studies. Halvorsen and Heyerdahl (2006) defined their outcome groups according to attitudes toward eating based on EDE assessment and DSM-IV criteria. Nilson and Hagglof (2005) defined recovery as no longer fulfilling DSM-III-R criteria. Wentz *et al.* (2005) used the modified Morgan–Russell assessment schedule and the Global Assessment of Functioning Scale (GAF). Deter *et al.* (2005) used the unmodified Morgan and Russell criteria and the Deter-Hertzog criteria. Holtkamp *et al.* (2005b) used the modified Morgan and Russell outcome classification system. A further problem in the latter study is the apparently interchangeable use of the terms 'symptoms', 'features' and 'personality traits'.

Although it is difficult to interpret these findings, given the many different criteria for defining outcome, a number of studies have attempted to define risk factors. Deter *et al.* (2005) focused on predictive factors and suggested that good outcome is predicted by younger onset, few psychological and social symptoms (as measured by psychological and social items in the Anorexia Nervosa Symptom Score (ANSS) clinical rating scale), and normal serum albumin and serum creatinine levels. With regard to age at onset, Nilson and Hagglof (2005) obtained contrasting findings. They found that children aged 10–13 years at first admission had significantly lower recovery rates than patients aged 14–17 years at first admission. Wentz *et al.* (2005) found that a history of child sexual abuse was not a risk factor for development of eating disorders.

Finally, there is some evidence that the mortality rate for AN has decreased. For example, Lindblad *et al.* (2006) found a decrease from 4.4% to 1.3 % between cohorts hospitalized during 1977–1981 and 1987–1991.

Summary of important findings and areas of interest

There is an increasing focus on the need to establish reliable and valid instruments for children and adolescents, and an acknowledgment of the importance of parental reports. The prevalence of eating disorders in adolescents might be underestimated, and ethnic differences may partly explain this. Physical complications in this age group are common, and the reduction in bone density is of particular concern. Levels of comorbidity are high, and the frequency of significant neuropsychological deficits and regional cerebral hypometabolism lends support to the view that at least some cases of AN in this age group have a neurodevelopmental substrate. Dependence upon weight or BMI and self-report of menstruation to determine changes in management or to define outcome has no scientific basis, and more valid and reliable criteria are required.

Treatments remain relatively ineffective. Medication has very little part to play, and patients evaluate treatment programs more positively when weight, shape and eating are not the sole focus, and when underlying problems such as low self-esteem or depressive thoughts are addressed.

Despite the increasing number of studies of family-based treatments, convincing evidence of their long-term value is lacking, not least because of major methodological flaws in nearly all of these studies. However, it is clear that family members should be viewed as a resource, and not as a focus of pathology.

The differences between reports with regard to the definitions of remission and recovery make it extremely difficult to draw any useful conclusions about outcome. Some reports use very generous criteria to define good outcome (e.g. 85% of ideal body weight as the only determinant). Unsurprisingly, the more stringent the criteria, the poorer the reported outcome. Previous reports that early-onset AN has a good prognosis have no convincing evidence base.

Clinical implications

A number of key issues arise. Comorbidity is common and needs to be assessed and treated. Neuropsychological deficits appear to be even more common, and a neuropsychological assessment should be routine. Within the physical domain, brain tumors should always be considered as an explanation for food avoidance and weight loss. Bone density should always be assessed, as a reduction in bone density (and even osteoporosis) is common. There are many other physical complications of weight loss that should be borne in mind. The use of target weights is not supported by empirical evidence, and given the unreliability of weight as a measure, decisions should never be made on the basis of weight or BMI alone. Self-reporting of menstruation is also unreliable, and should not be used when making any decisions about treatment.

There is no support for the use of psychotropic medication, and the use of bisphosphonates for the treatment of osteoporosis in this age group is absolutely contraindicated, even in clinical trials.

Parents should be actively included in the treatment program, and there should be a particular emphasis on enhancing family strengths, rather than on pathology. As far as possible AN should be managed in the naturalistic context of home life rather than the clinical setting of an inpatient ward. Multi-family therapy is becoming increasingly popular with both clinicians and families.

Future directions

More focus is required on the similarities and differences between the various child and adolescent eating disorder populations (e.g. boys versus girls, children from different cultural backgrounds) There is also a continued need to clarify differences between the younger population and adults with eating disorders, given a common tendency to extrapolate from the latter to the former. There is a pressing need for better designed treatment studies with larger samples, appropriate control and comparison groups, longer follow-up periods and standardized outcome criteria. Evaluations are required of 'naturalistic' treatments – that is, treatments which are not manualized, which tend to include combinations of approaches, and which are conducted in non-research-based clinics. There is an emerging trend away from the over-dependence of clinicians and researchers on weight as the key determinant of progress and outcome, and future studies should attempt to provide empirical support for this seemingly more realistic approach.

References

(References included from the targeted review years are preceded by one asterisk. References preceded by three asterisks are of particular significance. The significance is explained by a short commentary following the complete reference.)

*Abraham SF, Pettigrew B, Boyd C, Russell J and Taylor A (2005) Usefulness of amenorrhea in the diagnoses of eating disorder patients. *Journal of Psychosomatic Obstetrics and Gynaecology*, **26**: 211–15.

*Bass S, Saxon L, Corral A-M, Rodda C, Strauss B, Reidpath D *et al.* (2005) Near normalisation of lumbar spine bone density in young women with osteopenia recovered from adolescent onset anorexia nervosa – a longitudinal study. *Journal of Paediatric Endocrinology*, **18**: 897–907.

*Bergh C, Osgood M, Alters D, Maletz L, Leon M and Sodersten P (2006) How effective is family therapy for the treatment of anorexia nervosa? *European Eating Disorders Review*, **14**: 371–6.

*Binford RB, La Grange D and Jellar CC (2005) Eating disorders examination versus eating disorders examination-questionnaire in adolescents with full and partial-syndrome bulimia. *International Journal of Eating Disorders*, **37**: 44–9.

*Blinder BJ, Cumella EJ and Sanathara VA (2006) Psychiatric comorbidities of female inpatients with eating disorders. *Psychosomatic Medicine*, **68**: 454–62.

*Compston J, McConachie C, Stott C, Hannon R, Kaptoge S, Debiram I. *et al.* (2006) Changes in bone mineral density and biochemical markers of bone turnover during weight gain in adolescents with anorexia nervosa – a one-year prospective study. *Osteoporosis International*, **17**: 77–84.

*Cook-Darzens S, Doyen C, Falissard B and Mouren M-C (2005) Self-perceived family functioning in 40 French families of anorexic adolescents: implications for therapy. *European Eating Disorders Review*, **13**: 223–36.

*Couturier J and Lock J (2006a) Do supplementary items on the eating disorder examination improve the assessment of adolescents with anorexia nervosa? *International Journal of Eating Disorders*, **39**: 426–33.

***Couturier J and Lock J (2006b) What is recovery in adolescent anorexia nervosa? *International Journal of Eating Disorders*, **39**: 550–55.

***Couturier J and Lock J (2006c) What is remission in adolescent anorexia nervosa? A review of various conceptualizations and quantitative analysis. *International Journal of Eating Disorders*, **39**: 175–83.

These two papers show how outcome criteria differ enormously between studies, and consequently so do the reported outcomes. The findings illustrate the importance of using standardized outcome criteria across studies.

*Davis C, Blackmore E, Katzman DK and Fox J (2005) Female adolescents with anorexia nervosa and their parents: a case–control study of exercise attitudes and behaviours. *Psychological Medicine,* **35**: 377–86.

*Dennis K, Le Grange D and Bremer J (2006) Olanzapine use in adolescent anorexia nervosa. *Eating and Weight Disorders,* **11**: 53–6.

*Deter HC, Schelberg D, Kopp W, Friedrich HC and Herzog W (2005) Predictability of a favourable outcome in anorexia nervosa. *European Psychiatry,* **20**: 165–72.

Duchesne M, Mattos P, Fontenelle LF, Veiga H, Rizo L and Appolinario JC (2004) Neuropsychology of eating disorders: a systematic review of the literature. *Revista Brasileira de Psiquiatria,* **26**: 107–17.

*Eisenberg ME, Neumark-Sztainer D and Paxton SJ (2006) Five-year change in body satisfaction among adolescents. *Journal of Psychosomatic Research,* **61**: 521–7.

Eisler I (2005) The empirical and theoretical base of family therapy and multiple family day therapy for adolescent anorexia nervosa. *Journal of Family Therapy,* **27**: 104–31.

***Fairburn C (2005) Evidence-based treatment of anorexia nervosa. *International Journal of Eating Disorders,* **37**: S26–30.

This is a scholarly and critical review of treatment studies which shows that there is no convincing evidence that family-based treatments are a particularly effective therapy for adolescents with eating disorders. All of the studies to date have been too methodologically flawed to allow useful conclusions to be drawn, and it is not clear from these studies whether any beneficial effects are due to family involvement.

*Favaro A, Tenconi E and Santonastaso P (2006) Perinatal factors and the risk of developing anorexia nervosa and bulimia nervosa. *Archives of General Psychiatry,* **63**: 82–8.

*Fleminger S (2005) A model for the treatment of eating disorders of adolescents in a specialised centre in the Netherlands. *Journal of Family Therapy,* **27**: 147–57.

*Fowler L, Blackwell A, Jaffa A, Palmer R, Robbins TW, Sahakian BJ *et al.* (2005) Profile of neurocognitive impairments associated with female in-patients with anorexia nervosa. *Psychological Medicine,* **36**: 517–27.

*Gila A, Castro J, Cesena J and Toro J (2005) Anorexia nervosa in male adolescents: body image, eating attitudes and psychological traits. *Journal of Adolescent Health,* **36**: 221–6.

*Golden N, Iglesias E, Jacobson M, Carey D, Meyer W, Schebendach J *et al.* (2005) Alendroate for the treatment of osteopenia in anorexia nervosa – a randomised, double-blind, placebo-controlled trial. *Journal of Clinical Endocrinology and Metabolism,* **90**: 3179–85.

*Granillo T, Jones-Rodriguez G and Carvajal SC (2005) Prevalence of eating disorders in Latina adolescents: associations with substance use and other correlates. *Journal of Adolescent Health,* **36**: 214–20.

Hagenah U and Vloet T (2005) Parent psycho-education groups in the treatment of adolescents with eating disorders. *Praxis der Kinderpsychologie und Kinderpsychiatrie,* **54**: 303–17.

*Halvorsen I and Heyerdahl S (2006) Girls with anorexia nervosa as young adults: personality, self-esteem, and life satisfaction. *International Journal of Eating Disorders,* **39**: 285–93.

*Holtkamp K, Konrad K, Kaiser N, Ploynes Y, Heussen N, Grzella I. *et al.* (2005a) A retrospective study of SSRI treatment in adolescent anorexia nervosa. *Journal of Psychiatric Research*, **39**: 303–10.

*Holtkamp K, Muller B, Heussen N, Remschmidt H and Herpertz-Dahlmann B (2005b) Depression, anxiety and obsessionality in long-term recovered patients with adolescent-onset anorexia nervosa. *European Child and Adolescent Psychiatry*, **14**: 106–10.

*Honey A and Halse C (2006) The specifics of coping: parents of daughters with anorexia nervosa. *Qualitative Health Research*, **16**: 611–29.

*Honig P (2005) A multi-family group programme as part of an inpatient service for adolescents with a diagnosis of anorexia nervosa. *Clinical Child Psychology and Psychiatry*, **10**: 465–75.

*Imfeld C and Imfeld T (2005) Eating disorders – dental aspects. *Schweizer Monatsschrift fur Zahnmedizin*, **115**: 1163–71.

*Konstantynowicz J, Kadziela-Olech H and Kaczmarski M (2005) Depression in anorexia nervosa – a risk factor for osteopenia. *Journal of Clinical Endocrinology and Metabolism*, **90**: 5382–5.

Landis B, Richter M, Dojcinovic I and Hugentobler M (2006) Osteonecrosis of the jaw after treatment with bisphosphonates. *British Medical Journal*, **333**: 982–3.

***Lask B, Bryant-Waugh R, Wright F, Campbell M, Willoughby K and Waller G (2005a) Family physician consultation patterns indicate high risk for early-onset anorexia nervosa. *International Journal of Eating Disorders*, **38**: 269–72.
This study shows that just one consultation with a family physician about weight, shape or eating concerns reliably predicts the emergence of AN within 12 months.

*Lask B, Gordon I, Christie D, Chowdhury U and Watkins B (2005b) Functional neuroimaging in early-onset anorexia nervosa. *International Journal of Eating Disorders*, **37**: S49–51.

*Lee HY, Lee EL, Pathy P and Chan YC (2005) Anorexia nervosa in Singapore: an eight-year retrospective study. *Singapore Medical Journal*, **46**: 275.

*Le Grange D and Lock J (2005) The dearth of psychological treatment studies for anorexia nervosa. *International Journal of Eating Disorders*, **37**: 79–91.

*Le Grange D and Schmidt U (2005) The treatment of adolescents with bulimia nervosa. *Journal of Mental Health*, **14**: 587–97.

*Le Grange D, Binford R and Loeb K (2005) Manualised family-based treatment for anorexia nervosa: a case series. *Journal of the American Academy of Child and Adolescent Psychiatry*, **44**: 41–6.

*Lindblad F, Lindberg L and Hjern A (2006) Improved survival in adolescent patients with anorexia nervosa: a comparison of two Swedish national cohorts of female inpatients. *American Journal of Psychiatry*, **163**: 1433–5.

*Lock J (2005) Adjusting cognitive behavior therapy for adolescents with bulimia nervosa: results of a case series. *American Journal of Psychotherapy*, **59**: 267–81.

*Lock J, Agras S, Bryson S and Kraemer H (2005) A comparison of short- and long-term family therapy for adolescent anorexia nervosa. *Journal of the American Academy of Child and Adolescent Psychiatry*, **44**: 632–9.

*Lock J, Couturier J and Agras S (2006a) Comparison of long-term outcomes in adolescents with anorexia nervosa treated with family therapy. *Journal of the American Academy of Child and Adolescent Psychiatry*, **45**: 666–72.

*Lock J, Couturier J, Bryson S and Agras S (2006b) Predictors of drop out and remission in family therapy for adolescent anorexia nervosa in a randomised clinical trial. *International Journal of Eating Disorders*, **39**: 639–47.

McDermott B, Forbes D, Harris C, McCormack J and Gibbon P (2006) Non-eating disorders psychopathology in children and adolescents with eating disorders: implications for malnutrition and symptom severity. *Journal of Psychosomatic Research*, **60**: 257–61.

*May A, Kim J, McHale S and Crouter A (2006) Parent–adolescent relationships and the development of weight concerns from early to late adolescence. *International Journal of Eating Disorders*, **39**: 729–40.

*Nilson K and Hagglof B (2005) Long-term follow-up of adolescent-onset anorexia nervosa in northern Sweden. *European Eating Disorders Review*, **13**: 89–100.

***Offord A, Turner H and Cooper M (2006) Adolescent inpatient treatment for anorexia nervosa: a qualitative study exploring young adults' retrospective views of treatment and discharge. *European Eating Disorder Review*, **14**: 377–87.

This study focuses on what patients find helpful and unhelpful in treatment for anorexia nervosa. The findings are in line with the stances of motivational therapy, in which there is promotion of respect for the patient's views, and of collaborative treatment.

*Olivares J, Vazquez M, Fleta J, Moreno LA, Perez-Gonzalez JM and Bueno M (2005) Cardiac findings in adolescents with anorexia nervosa at diagnosis and weight restoration. *European Journal of Pediatrics*, **164**: 383–6.

*Ott S (2005) Alendroate in anorexia nervosa (letter to editor). *Journal of Clinical Endocrinology and Metabolism*, **90**: 5508.

*Paulson-Karlsson G, Nevonen L and Engstrom I (2006) Treatment satisfaction. *Journal of Family Therapy*, **28**: 293–306.

*Peebles R, Wilson J and Lock J (2006) How do children with eating disorders differ from adolescents with eating disorders at initial evaluation? *Journal of Adolescent Health*, **39**: 800–5.

*Perkins S, Schmidt U, Eisler I, Treasure J, Yi I., Winn S et al. (2005) Why do adolescents with bulimia nervosa choose not to involve their parents in treatment? *European Child and Adolescent Psychiatry*, **14**: 376–85.

*Pieters G, Hulstijn W, Vandereycken W, Maas Y, Probst M, Peuskens J et al. (2005) Fast psychomotor functioning in anorexia nervosa: effects of weight restoration. *Journal of Clinical and Experimental Neuropsychology*, **27**: 931–42.

*Ravaldi C, Vannacci A, Bolognesi E, Mancini S, Faravelli C and Ricca V (2006) Gender role, eating disorder symptoms, and body image concern in ballet dancers. *Journal of Psychosomatic Research*, **61**: 529–35.

*Rhodes P, Baillie A, Brown J and Madden S (2005) Parental efficacy in the family-based treatment of anorexia: preliminary development of the Parent Versus Anorexia Scale (PVA). *European Eating Disorders Review*, **13**: 399–405.

*Rodriguez-Cano T, Beato-Fernandes L and Belmonte-Llario A (2005) New contributions to the prevalence of eating disorders in Spanish adolescents: detection of false negatives. *European Psychiatry*, **20**: 173–8.

*Rohrer T, Fahlbusch R, Buchfelder M and Dorr H (2006) Craniopharyngioma in a female adolescent presenting with symptoms of anorexia nervosa. *Klinishe Padiatre*, **218**: 67–71.

*Roots P, Hawker J and Gowers S (2006) The use of target weights in the inpatient treatment of adolescent anorexia nervosa. *European Eating Disorders Review*, **14**: 323–8.

*Ruuska J, Kaltiala-Heino R, Rantanen P and Koivisto AM (2005) Are there differences in the attitudinal body image between adolescent anorexia nervosa and bulimia nervosa? *Eating and Weight Disorders*, **10**: 98–106.

*Schapman-Williams AM, Lock J and Couturier J (2006) Cognitive-behavioral therapy for adolescents with binge eating syndromes: a case series. *International Journal of Eating Disorders*, **39**: 252–5.

*Scholz M, Rix M, Scholz K, Gantchev K and Thomke V (2005) Multiple family therapy for anorexia nervosa: concepts, experiences and results. *Journal of Family Therapy*, **27**: 132–41.

*Serpell L, Hirani V, Willoughby K, Neiderman M and Lask B (2006) Personality or pathology? Obsessive-compulsive symptoms in children and adolescents with anorexia nervosa. *European Eating Disorders Review*, **14**: 404–13.

*Strumia R (2005) Dermatological signs in patients with eating disorders. *American Journal of Clinical Dermatology*, **6**: 165–73.

*Swenne I, Belfrage E, Thurfjell B and Engstrom I (2005) Accuracy of reported weight and menstrual status in teenage girls with eating disorders. *International Journal of Eating Disorders*, **38**: 375–9,

*Tareen A, Hodes M and Rangel L (2005) Non-fat-phobic anorexia nervosa in British South Asian adolescents. *International Journal of Eating Disorders*, **37**: 161–5.

*Ulger Z, Gurses D, Ozyurek A and Arikan C (2006) Follow-up of cardiac abnormalities in female adolescents with anorexia nervosa after re-feeding. *Acta Cardiologica*, **61**: 43–9.

*Watkins B, Frampton I, Lask B and Bryant-Waugh R (2005) Reliability and validity of the child version of the Eating Disorder Examination: a preliminary investigation. *International Journal of Eating Disorders*, **38**: 183–7.

*Wentz E, Gillberg IC, Gillberg C and Rastam M (2005) Fertility and history of sexual abuse at 10-year follow-up of adolescent-onset anorexia nervosa. *International Journal of Eating Disorders*, **37**: 294–8.

*Whitney J, Murray J, Gavan K, Todd G, Whitaker W and Treasure J (2005) Experience of caring for someone with anorexia nervosa: qualitative study. *British Journal of Psychiatry*, **187**: 444–9.

*Zucker N, Marcus M and Bulik C (2006) A group parent-training programme: a novel approach for eating disorder management. *Eating and Weight Disorders*, **11**: 78–82.

9

Treatment of bulimia nervosa

G Terence Wilson and Katie Bannon

Abstract

Objectives of review. The aim of this review is to highlight important developments in the treatment of bulimia nervosa (BN).

Summary of recent findings. The current literature reflects the following findings. Manual-based cognitive–behavioural therapy (CBT) is currently the first choice of treatment. Recent enhancements of CBT are likely to produce even more successful outcomes. A guided self-help adaptation of CBT has begun to yield promising results. Utilization and dissemination of evidence-based treatment are still poor. Early response to treatment may be a robust predictor of outcome in the use of antidepressant medication. In the USA, residential treatment is growing in popularity, embraces a kaleidoscopic mix of interventions, and lacks empirical support for its effectiveness.

Future directions. The development of even more effective treatments that apply to a diverse range of different patients, including adolescents, remains a research priority. Innovative research is needed to improve training in evidence-based treatment and to evaluate more effective means of disseminating research findings to routine clinical practice.

Introduction

This review focuses on the clinical literature published in 2005 and 2006 on the treatment of bulimia nervosa (BN).

Literature review

American Psychiatric Association Practice Guideline for Treatment of Patients with Eating Disorders (Third Edition)

The most recent edition of the American Psychiatric Association (APA) Practice Guideline is little changed from the second edition (published in 2000). Its strengths include a comprehensive summary of the defining clinical features, epidemiology, etiology, course and treatment of the full range of eating disorders. The guideline provides up-to-date and practical information on the medical complications of eating disorders and their management. The summary and analysis of pharmacological therapy are comprehensive, current and incisive. However, despite the useful information that it provides for practitioners in many areas, the guideline is not without problems.

The limitations of the APA guideline can be highlighted by comparing it with the National Institute for Health and Clinical Excellence (NICE) guideline (National Institute for Health and Clinical Excellence 2004) from the UK. Suffice it here to highlight a few of the significant differences between the two guidelines (for a fuller discussion, see Wilson and Shafran 2005). The first difference concerns methodological adequacy. The APA guideline provides 'three categories of endorsement' of its various recommendations. These categories, based on the 'level of clinical confidence', are as follows:

I   recommended with substantial clinical confidence
II   recommended with moderate clinical confidence
III may be recommended on the basis of individual circumstances.

The guideline does not detail the scientific criteria that are used to make these categorical evaluations. Rather, it blends science with subjective clinical judgment without consistently distinguishing between the two (Wilson and Agras 2001). The NICE guideline provides recommendations that are based on an interdisciplinary, quantitative and rigorous process.

Secondly, the APA guideline favors subjective judgment in the selection of treatments in clinical practice. It recommends that treatment 'be chosen on the basis of a comprehensive evaluation of the individual patient, considering cognitive and psychological development, psychodynamic issues, cognitive style, comorbid psychopathology, patient preferences and family situation' (American Psychiatric Assocation 2006, p. 19). Moreover, this recommendation is given a rating of I. As Wilson and Shafran (2005) point out, 'A problem with this recommendation is that at present we cannot identify pretreatment characteristics that reliably predict outcome and enable therapists to match treatments to patients. The more general problem is its reliance on subjective clinical judgment which, among other limitations, allows the uncritical use of personally preferred treatments rather than choosing the most effective method' (p. 80). In their survey of the types of psychological treatment that are provided for eating-disordered patients in Canada, von Ranson and Robinson (2006) documented that clinicians based their treatment on their personal clinical experiences rather than on research. They aptly noted that 'Although this desire to tailor treatments to individual needs has face validity, it may be misguided. Reliance on clinical judgment is at odds with a body of research on clinical versus actuarial prediction indicating that, on the whole, actuarial methods are superior, in part, because clinicians tend to identify too many exceptions to effective rules' (pp. 32–3). The increasing focus on identifying moderators of treatment effects and mediators of change in controlled research represents an important step towards providing practitioners with much needed information about matching interventions to specific problems.

The NICE guideline provides a better balance between scientific research and clinical judgment. The latter is decisive when research is lacking and when an evidence-based 'treatment needs to be adapted to the niceties of an individual or when an alternative approach is needed. On the other hand, where sufficient evidence exists to allow general recommendation (e.g. in bulimia nervosa, BN), the best practice must be to implement the treatment that enjoys the most empirical support rather than invoke subjective judgment' (Wilson and Shafran 2005, p. 81).

Thirdly, the APA guideline is uncritically inclusive of psychological therapies for which there is little if any empirical support. For example, it states that 'using psychodynamic interventions in conjunction with CBT and other psychotherapies may yield better global outcomes (e.g. comorbidity and quality or life) versus binge eating and purging' (p. 19). This assertion is given a rating of II despite the absence of controlled research. Relying on uncontrolled, naturalistic reports of treatment outcome can never substitute for controlled evaluations of effectiveness. It is difficult, if not impossible, to know precisely what treatments are used in clinical practice and what effects they have. Specification of and empirical research on 'treatment as usual' remains a priority.

Fourthly, the APA guideline would appear to miss an important opportunity to promote the dissemination of evidence-based treatment. It is well documented that evidence-based treatment such as cognitive–behavioral therapy (CBT) for BN is not widely adopted in routine clinical practice in the USA. The APA guideline does conclude that CBT 'is the most effective intervention' for BN, and does imply that given 'qualified therapists', CBT is the initial treatment of choice (p. 20). However, the guideline does not make a clear-cut recommendation that therapists be trained in this approach and that it be implemented as the recommended treatment. Rather, the guideline notes that clinicians '*may benefit* (our italics) from acquainting themselves with CBT treatment manuals ...' (p. 83).

Cognitive–behavioral therapy (CBT)

Predictors of response to CBT

Previous reviews have concluded that pretreatment patient characteristics that reliably predict treatment outcome have proved to be elusive. Although it is widely assumed that borderline personality disorder is a negative predictor of outcome (e.g. American Psychiatric Association 2006), the evidence is conflicting

(National Institute for Health and Clinical Excellence 2004). Moreover, Grilo *et al.* (2007) have replicated previous findings which show that the natural course of BN does not appear to be influenced by the presence or severity of co-occurring personality disorder psychopathology, including borderline personality disorder. Given this context, the findings of a study by Butryn *et al.* (2006) are of particular interest. In a re-analysis of the data of Agras *et al.* (2000), they showed that weight suppression (the difference between a patient's highest adult weight ever and their present weight) predicted drop-out rate as well as remission from binge eating and purging at post-treatment. Butryn *et al.* (2006) conclude that patients with high weight suppression will be more reluctant to abandon dietary restraint that has been shown to mediate, at least in part, the maintenance and modification of BN. In speculating as to how CBT might be modified to address the putative significance of weight suppression, they suggest that treatment would need to target the belief that normal eating would necessarily lead to weight gain. Such a strategy has always been a core feature of manual-based CBT for BN (Fairburn *et al.* 1993). On average, patients do not gain weight as a result of CBT that eliminates binge eating and purging. As manual-based CBT has evolved, it has focused on the balance between acceptance and change (Wilson 2005), and the importance of developing domains of self-evaluation and self-worth other than body shape and weight (Fairburn *et al.* in press). These advances would seem to directly address the concern about possible weight gain expressed by patients with high weight suppression.

Improving the efficacy of manual-based CBT

One of the recommended strategies for improving the success rate of manual-based CBT for BN is to individualize treatment to a greater degree than has previously been the case (Wilson 2005). The best example of this strategy to date is the enhanced CBT of Fairburn *et al.* (2003).

Ghaderi (2006) completed a preliminary study of what he called individualized CBT versus standardized CBT. The latter consisted of the Fairburn *et al.* (1993) manual. The individualized treatment used the manual as a basis, but was modified according to functional analyses of individual patients. This resulted in a more intensive focus on three particular mechanisms, namely interpersonal difficulties, affect regulation and increased acceptance of emotions and thoughts. The consistency with the enhanced CBT of Fairburn *et al.* (2003) is notable. In order to use functional analysis in a manner that was replicable and less subject to criticism of its possible idiosyncratic nature, Ghaderi (2006) adopted the guidelines of logical functional analysis as described by Hayes and Follette (1992).

The results of this study showed that both treatments produced substantial improvement at post-treatment and at a six-month follow-up. The individualized treatment was significantly superior on some measures, including the number of weeks of abstinence from binge eating. As Ghaderi (2006) notes, the lack of statistical power makes it difficult to interpret the overall findings.

However, the research should encourage future studies with a sufficient sample size and other methodological improvements.

A systematic focus on interpersonal issues has long been advocated as a means of improving therapeutic efficacy (Wilson 1996), and is a significant component of the enhanced CBT approach of Fairburn *et al.* (2003). Binford *et al.* (2006) found that social support seeking significantly predicted maintenance of therapeutic improvement at a 6-month follow-up, and they recommend this form of coping as a potentially effective means of preventing relapse.

Treatment of adolescents

It is important to address BN in adolescence, because the disorder usually begins around puberty, indicating the role of developmental factors in its onset (Commission on Adolescent Eating Disorders 2005). Moreover, BN and related eating disorders in adolescence are also risk factors for a variety of other physical and mental disorders during early adulthood (Commission on Adolescent Eating Disorders 2005). Lock (2005) and Wilson and Sysko (2006) have described adaptations of CBT that take into account the specific developmental features of adolescence. In the first controlled trial of its kind, Schmidt *et al.* (2007) compared family therapy (based on the Maudsley model) with guided self-help (GSH) based on cognitive–behavioral principles in the treatment of adolescents with BN or eating disorders not otherwise specified (EDNOS). GSH resulted in a more rapid response, greater acceptability and lower cost than family therapy.

Dissemination of CBT

The relative lack of availability of adequately administered CBT for BN in routine clinical practice has been well documented. Patients are not benefiting from advances in clinical research. One of the various reasons for this is the lack of appropriate training in graduate psychology programs in North America (Wilson *et al.* 2007), but the problem is not lack of interest on the part of clinicians (e.g. von Ranson and Robinson 2006). We face two challenges in this regard.

First, we need innovative research on how to more effectively train sufficient numbers of skilled therapists. Referring to psychological therapy as a whole, Holloway and Neufeldt (1995) observed that 'Just as supervision demands of trainees a systematic and deliberate delivery of treatment to the client, so it must be demanded of supervisors that they deliver the requisite skills to the trainee. ... To accomplish this goal, researchers must now devise clear methods of training, standardized manuals for its delivery, and empirical studies that will test its effectiveness as a contributing component in psychotherapy training' (p. 208). Yet the literature on supervision and training is consistent in noting the absence of evidence for the effectiveness of different formats of supervision and clinical training. Looking to the future, we can anticipate that the tools of instructional design and technology will be harnessed to translate current text-based, manual-based therapies into 'media-rich, interactive and web-based applications'

(Weingardt 2004). Research on the dissemination of CBT-based interventions for eating disorders via the use of computer-based interventions is under way (Schmidt and Grover 2007).

Secondly, we need to modify and refine existing treatments so that they can be more readily disseminated by a wide range of mental health professionals. As Hayes *et al.* (2006) have argued with regard to empirically supported, multi-component treatments in general, the goal here is to identify basic mechanisms and principles of behavior change that will make it easier to teach essential treatment strategies.

Dieting reconsidered

Burton and Stice (2006) compared their six-session, group-based Healthy Weight program with a waiting-list control condition in the treatment of full and sub-threshold BN patients. In the latter, the average frequency of binge eating was only once a week. The treatment program was significantly more effective than the control condition, resulting in remission rates of 16% and 35% at post-treatment and three-month follow-up, respectively. Compared with the controls, the treatment program was also superior in decreasing healthcare utilization over the full course of the study, and in reducing BMI.

Burton and Stice (2006) concluded that their treatment results compare favorably with manual-based CBT, and reported that the average per-session effect size was higher than in CBT. They also observed that the treatment might be well suited to the minority of BN patients who are overweight or obese. Perhaps more importantly – and controversially – they interpreted the findings as showing that dieting does not play a pivotal role in the maintenance or modification of BN. This interpretation is based on their demonstration of both weight loss and decreased bulimic behavior. It should also be noted that the findings are consistent with other recent experimental studies of dietary restraint theory (e.g. Stice *et al.* 2005).

Burton and Stice (2006) distinguished their treatment from manual-based CBT as follows: 'What differentiates this program from CBT is that weight management is encouraged, rather than discouraged. In fact, facilitators utilize participant drive for thinness as a motivator to achieve a slim but healthy figure through healthy means. In other words, unlike CBT, this intervention promotes caloric restriction and leaves the pursuit of the thin ideal intact' (p. 1730). However, the differences might not be that pronounced. First, the weight loss, although statistically significant, was minimal (a BMI fraction of 0.23). Secondly, the Healthy Weight program encourages healthy (regular?) and moderate eating designed to produce a 'slight' negative energy balance. The overlap with manual-based CBT is clear. However, leaving the 'thin ideal intact' does differ from the goal of CBT. Outcomes for measures of body shape and weight concerns were not reported. Other evidence indicates that failure to alter body shape and weight concerns is linked to poorer long-term outcome (Fairburn *et al.*, in press). The findings of Burton and Stice (2006) should encourage replication and further analysis.

Self-help strategies

Efficient and focused self-help interventions based on the principles of CBT provide a potentially important means of disseminating this treatment approach more widely. Evidence exists that GSH – which combines a self-help manual with a limited number of brief 'therapy' sessions – is effective for at least subsets of adult patients. In Australia, Banasiak *et al.* (2005) showed that practitioners in a primary care setting who were trained and supervised in GSH obtained significantly superior results to a delayed treatment control condition. The results were maintained at a six-month follow-up, and rivalled the outcomes of more standard manual-based CBT. Whether these findings could be generalized to different clinical settings and other therapists is questionable. The physicians in this Australian study were committed to treating eating-disordered patients, and spent a significant amount of time administering GSH. The level of training and expertise necessary to successfully administer GSH is unclear, although it seems safe to conclude that unsupervised mental health providers with minimal training are unlikely to be effective (Sysko and Walsh 2007).

A recent study from Sweden provides further evidence for the possible efficacy of GSH (Ljotsson *et al.* 2007). BN patients were assigned the Fairburn (1995) self-help manual and, via email contact with graduate clinical psychology students, received systematic guidance in completing the program. Patients were also given access to an online discussion forum. All patient contact was supervised by a clinical psychologist. Again the results were comparable with those obtained using formal manual-based CBT. The importance of personalized feedback on patient progress was demonstrated in a study in which patients with either BN or EDNOS were treated with GSH (Schmidt *et al.* 2006). Patients who received personalized feedback during the trial showed greater improvement on measures of vomiting and dietary restraint than those who did not receive such feedback.

In their data-based review of the self-help literature for eating disorders, Perkins *et al.* (2006) concluded that GSH may be useful as a first intervention in a stepped-care framework, and 'may have potential as an alternative to formal therapist-delivered psychological therapy'. The authors of this Cochrane Review called for larger, well-controlled studies of self-help that include health economic analyses. The first major study of the cost-effectiveness of GSH with adults within a stepped-care framework has yielded encouraging results (Crow *et al.* 2006). GSH resulted in a substantially lower cost per effectively treated patient than regular CBT. Similarly, as noted above, Schmidt *et al.* (2007) showed that GSH for adolescents was as effective as family therapy, and involved significantly less cost.

Pharmacotherapy

Rapid response (within the first five to eight sessions) has been shown to be a robust predictor of short- and longer-term outcome in manual-based CBT, a finding that has significant theoretical and practical implications (Fairburn *et al.*

2004). Walsh *et al.* (2006) have uncovered a related finding with regard to desipramine. Patients who failed to respond to this antidepressant were reliably identified by their failure to respond (a 50% reduction in binge eating or vomiting) by the end of week two of treatment. Replication of this preliminary study with fluoxetine, which is more widely used and is approved by the FDA for treatment of BN, is required.

One of the newer drugs that has attracted attention as a putative treatment for eating disorders is the anticonvulsant topiramate. The APA guideline cautions that, owing to serious side-effects, this drug should only be used when other medications have proved ineffective. The guideline also notes that topiramate results in weight loss which would be 'problematic for normal or underweight individuals' (p. 20). The prudent APA guideline is in contrast to the uncritical advocacy of topiramate in the literature (e.g. Arnone 2005). Consider, for example, a brief double-blind study by Nickel *et al.* (2005), who concluded that the drug was safe and effective. Part of their rationale for testing this drug was that antidepressants perform poorly in producing remission from binge eating and purging. However, they did not report remission rates – only reductions in frequency of symptoms, which were not particularly impressive. Moreover, they predictably obtained weight loss in BN patients whose mean pretreatment BMI was only 22.7.

Residential treatment

The APA guideline concludes that most BN patients do not require hospitalization. However, a survey by Frisch *et al.* (2006) found that residential treatment of individuals with anorexia nervosa (AN) and BN is 'a growing, variable and unregulated' business (p. 434). The average length of stay was 83 days, with an average cost per day of $956. It is impossible to distinguish between AN and BN in this survey, but either way the findings are troubling. Predictably, most programs reported 'an eclectic, integrative approach' to treatment (p. 437). More revealing is an analysis by Frisch *et al.* (2006) of the average amount of time spent each week on specific therapeutic interventions. In terms of minutes per week per patient, art and the 12-step approach were listed as 262 and 208 minutes, respectively. The comparable figures for CBT and dialectical behavior therapy (DBT) were 29 and 13 minutes, respectively – less than the figures for 'equine' and 'dance'! Frisch *et al.* (2006) call for empirical evaluations of the effectiveness of these high-priced programs.

Summary of findings

The APA guideline reaffirms previous reviews which have suggested that theory-driven, manual-based CBT for BN has the most empirical support. However, adequate graduate training in CBT is lacking, and the utilization and dissemination of manual-based CBT are unacceptably poor.

Guided self-help (GSH) based on CBT principles is an effective intervention for some BN patients. It appears to be cost-effective, and may facilitate wider dissemination of evidence-based treatment.

Antidepressant medication has a rapid effect that can be used to identify likely treatment failures. Residential treatments are growing in popularity, expensive and unregulated. There is currently no evidence of their efficacy.

Clinical implications

The APA guideline lends additional support to the use of manual-based CBT as the treatment of first choice. Individualizing the application of CBT within a theoretically coherent framework is likely to result in even more effective treatment. The enhanced CBT of Fairburn *et al.* (in press) provides the most systematic and comprehensive way of doing this.

CBT-guided self-help may be effective as an alternative to full CBT with a subset of patients, and is useful within a stepped-care framework. It is cost-effective, and its simpler and more focused nature might facilitate more widespread utilization of the approach.

There is a need for improved and more readily available clinical training in order to increase the number of therapists with expertise in the administration of evidence-based psychological treatment.

Rapid response treatment is a robust predictor of outcome in CBT, and may well serve the same function in treatment with antidepressant medication. This would enable therapists to identify likely failures and alter treatment protocols accordingly.

The distinction between healthy and dysfunctional dieting, and their roles in the maintenance and treatment of BN, both warrant detailed attention.

Future directions

The development of even more effective treatments is a research priority. It is also necessary to demonstrate the effectiveness of evidence-based treatments for a wider range of patients (e.g. adolescents, and patients with BN-like eating disorder not otherwise specified) than is currently the case. Finally, there is a need to improve the training of qualified therapists, and to promote greater utilization and dissemination of evidence-based treatments.

Acknowledgement

We are grateful to Carlos Grilo, PhD, for his comments on this review.

References

(References included from the targeted review years are preceded by one asterisk. References preceded by three asterisks are of particular significance. The significance is explained by a short commentary following the complete reference.)

Agras WS, Crow SJ, Halmi KA, Mitchell JE, Wilson GT and Kraemer H (2000) Outcome predictors for the cognitive-behavioral treatment of bulimia nervosa: data from a multisite study. *American Journal of Psychiatry* **157**: 1302–8.

American Psychiatric Association (2000) Practice guideline for the treatment of patients with eating disorders (second edition). *American Journal of Psychiatry*, **157 (Suppl. 1):** 1–39.

***American Psychiatric Association (2006) Practice guideline for treatment of patients with eating disorders (third edition). *American Journal of Psychiatry*, 163 **(Suppl. 7):** 4–54.

This is a comprehensive review of the clinical management and treatment of eating disorders. It lacks the methodological rigor of the NICE guideline, and is uncritically inclusive in recommending psychological therapies.

*Arnone D (2005) Review of the use of Topiramate for treatment of psychiatric disorders. *Annals of General Psychiatry*, **4:** 1–14.

*Banasiak SJ, Paxton SJ and Hay P (2005) Guided self-help for bulimia nervosa in primary care: a randomized controlled trial. *Psychological Medicine*, **35:** 1283–94.

*Binford RB, Mussell MP, Crosby RD, Peterson CB, Crow SJ and Mitchell JE (2005) Coping strategies in bulimia nervosa treatment: impact on outcome in group cognitive–behavioral therapy. *Journal of Consulting and Clinical Psychology*, **73:** 1089–96.

Burton E and Stice E (2006) Evaluation of a healthy-weight treatment program for bulimia nervosa: a preliminary randomized trial. *Behaviour Research and Therapy*, **44:** 1727–38.

Butryn ML, Lowe MR, Safer DL and Agras WS (2006) Weight suppression is a robust predictor of outcome in the cognitive–behavioral treatment of bulimia nervosa. *Journal of Abnormal Psychology*, **115:** 62–7.

***Commission on Adolescent Eating Disorders (2005) Eating disorders. In: Evans DL, Foa EB, Gur RE, Hendin H, O'Brien CP, Seligman MEP and Walsh BT, editors. *Treating and Preventing Adolescent Mental Health Disorders: what we know and what we don't know*. New York: Oxford University Press, Annenberg Foundation Trust at Sunnylands, and Annenberg Public Policy Center of the University of Pennsylvania.

This is a comprehensive and critical analysis of what we do and do not know about the development and treatment of eating disorders in adolescents. It is the best single source of information on this neglected area.

Crow S, Nyman JA, Agras WS, Halmi K, Fairburn CG and Mitchell J (2006) *Cost-effectiveness of stepped-care treatment for bulimia nervosa*. Paper presented at the Eating Disorders Research Society, Port Douglas, Australia, 31 August 2006.

Fairburn CG (1995) *Overcoming Binge Eating*. New York: Guilford Press.

Fairburn CG, Marcus MD and Wilson GT (1993) Cognitive behaviour therapy for binge eating and bulimia nervosa: a comprehensive treatment manual. In: Fairburn CG and Wilson GT, editors. *Binge Eating: nature, assessment and treatment*. New York: Guilford Press, pp. 361–404.

Fairburn CG, Cooper Z and Shafran R (2003) Cognitive behaviour therapy for eating disorders: a "transdiagnostic" theory and treatment. *Behaviour Research and Therapy*, **41:** 509–29.

Fairburn CG, Agras WS, Walsh BT, Wilson GT and Stice E (2004) Prediction of outcome in bulimia nervosa by early change in treatment. *American Journal of Psychiatry*, **161:** 2322–4.

Fairburn CG, Cooper Z, Shafran R and Wilson GT (in press) Eating disorders. In: Barlow DH, editor. *Clinical Handbook of Psychological Disorders* (4e). New York: Guilford Press.

*Frisch MJ, Herzog DB and Franko DL (2006) Residential treatment for eating disorders. *International Journal of Eating Disorders*, **39**: 434–42.

***Ghaderi A (2006) Does individualization matter? A randomized trial of standardized (focused) versus individualized (broad) cognitive behavior therapy for bulimia nervosa. *Behaviour Research and Therapy*, **44**: 273–88.

This is an initial study of the merits of tailoring manual-based CBT to individual patients. This approach strikes a good balance between evidence-based structure and clinical judgement and flexibility.

Grilo CM, Pagano ME, Skodol AE, Sanislow CA, McGlashan TH, Gunderson JG *et al.* (2007) Natural course of bulimia nervosa and of eating disorder not otherwise specified: 5-year prospective study of remissions, relapses, and the effects of personality disorder psychopathology. *Journal of Clinical Psychiatry*, **68**: 738–46.

Hayes SC and Follette WC (1992) Can functional analysis provide a substitute for syndromal classification? *Behavioral Assessment*, **14**: 345–65.

*Hayes SC, Luoma JB, Bond FW, Masuda A and Lillis J (2006) Acceptance and commitment therapy: model, processes and outcomes. *Behaviour Research and Therapy*, **44**: 1–25.

Holloway EL and Neufeldt SA (1995) Supervision: its contributions to treatment efficacy. *Journal of Consulting and Clinical Psychology*, **63**: 207–13.

Ljotsson B, Lundin C, Mitsell K, Carlbring P, Ramklint M and Ghaderi A (2007) Remote treatment of bulimia nervosa and binge eating disorder: a randomized trial of Internet-assisted cognitive behavioural therapy. *Behaviour Research and Therapy*, **45**: 649–61.

*Lock J (2005) Adjusting cognitive behavior therapy for adolescents with bulimia nervosa. *American Journal of Psychotherapy*, **59**: 267–81.

National Institute for Health and Clinical Excellence (2004) *Eating Disorders: core interventions in the treatment and management of anorexia nervosa, bulimia nervosa and related eating disorders*. London: NICE Clinical Guideline No 9, www.nice.org.uk

*Nickel C, Tritt K, Muehlbacher M, Pedrosa Gil F, Mitterlehner FO, Kaplan P *et al.* (2005) Topiramate treatment in bulimia nervosa patients: a randomized, double-blind, placebo-controlled trial. *International Journal of Eating Disorders*, **38**: 295–300.

***Perkins SJ, Murphy R, Schmidt U and Williams C (2006) Self-help and guided self-help for eating disorders. *Cochrane Database of Systematic Reviews*. Issue 3. Oxford: Update Software.

This is a searching review and analysis of the advantages and disadvantages of self-help approaches to treatment.

Schmidt U and Grover M (2007) Computer-based intervention for bulimia nervosa and binge eating. In: Latner JD, Wilson GT, editors. *Self-Help Approaches for Obesity and Eating Disorders: research and practice*. New York: Guilford Press.

Schmidt U, Landau S, Pombo-Carril MG, Bara-Carril N, Reid Y, Murray K *et al.* (2006) Does personalized feedback improve the outcome of cognitive-behavioural guided self-care in bulimia nervosa? A preliminary randomized controlled trial. *British Journal of Clinical Psychology*, **45**: 111–21.

Schmidt U, Lee S, Beecham J, Perkins S, Treasure J, Yi I *et al.* (2007) A randomized controlled trial of family therapy and cognitive behavior therapy guided self-care for adolescents with bulimia nervosa and related disorders. *American Journal of Psychiatry*, **164**: 591–8.

*Stice E, Presnell K, Groesz L and Shaw H (2005) Effects of a weight maintenance diet on bulimic pathology: an experimental test of the dietary restraint theory. *Health Psychology*, **24**: 402–12.

Sysko R and Walsh BT (2007) Guided self-help for bulimia nervosa. In: Latner JD, Wilson GT, editors. *Self-Help Approaches for Obesity and Eating Disorders: research and practice.* New York: Guilford Press.

***von Ranson K and Robinson K (2006) Who is providing what type of psychotherapy to eating disorder clients? A survey. *International Journal of Eating Disorders,* **39:** 27–34.

This is an informative and thoughtful analysis of a survey of practitioners in the community and the treatments that they provide. It highlights the dearth of adequate training in CBT and the relative lack of impact of research findings on clinical practice.

*Walsh BT, Sysko R and Parides MK (2006) Early response to desipramine among women with bulimia nervosa. *International Journal of Eating Disorders,* **39:** 72–5.

Weingardt KR (2004) The role of instructional design and technology in the dissemination of empirically supported manual-based therapies. *Clinical Psychology: Science and Practice,* **11:** 313–33.

Wilson GT (1996) Treatment of bulimia nervosa: when CBT fails. *Behaviour Research and Therapy,* **34:** 197–212.

*Wilson GT (2005) Psychological treatment of eating disorders. In: Nolen-Hoeksema S, editor. *Annual Review of Clinical Psychology. Volume 1.* Palo Alto, CA: Annual Reviews Inc.

Wilson GT and Agras WS (2001) Practice guidelines for treatment of eating disorders. *Behavior Therapy,* **32:** 219–34.

***Wilson GT and Shafran R (2005) Eating disorders guidelines from NICE. *Lancet,* **365:** 79–81.

This paper contrasts the methodological rigor and conceptual bases of the NICE guideline with those of the American Psychiatric Association guideline.

*Wilson GT and Sysko R (2006) Cognitive–behavioral therapy for adolescents with bulimia nervosa. *European Eating Disorders Review,* **14:** 8–16.

Wilson GT, Grilo C and Vitousek K (in press) Psychological treatment of eating disorders. *American Psychologist,* **62:** 199–216.

10

Treatment for anorexia nervosa

Kathleen Pike, Evelyn Attia and Amanda Joelle Brown

Abstract

Objectives of review. This review provides an overview and update of the empirical database for treatment of anorexia nervosa (AN) published subsequent to the previous summary in the 2006 edition of the *Annual Review of Eating Disorders*.

Summary of recent findings. The number of randomized controlled trials (RCTs) that have evaluated treatments for AN and been published during 2005 and 2006 is limited. However, recent studies contribute to a gradually expanding knowledge base regarding psychotherapy and medication for adolescents and adults with AN. The challenges inherent in conducting AN treatment research include the fact that full-syndrome AN is a relatively rare disorder, and individuals with AN are ambivalent about treatments that, by definition, aim to bring about weight restoration.

Future directions. Multi-site studies are needed in order to obtain adequate recruitment for successful RCTs. In addition, analyses of predictors and mediators of treatment outcome will be important components of future RCTs of AN treatments.

Introduction

Anorexia nervosa (AN) is a serious mental illness with mortality rates that are among the highest of any psychiatric illness. The development of new treatments has been identified by the National Institute of Mental Health (NIMH) Workshop on Anorexia Nervosa as a high priority (Agras *et al.* 2004). However, despite this research agenda and despite the long history of documenting the complexities of AN treatment in the clinical literature, establishing empirically based treatments for AN presents significant challenges for clinical researchers. In fact, for all phases of AN treatment and for all age groups, we have more questions than answers. Programmatic research in the treatment of AN is handicapped by the reality that full-syndrome AN is a relatively rare disorder and individuals with AN are ambivalent about treatments that, by definition, aim to help with weight restoration. Medical complications frequently mean that individuals have to withdraw from clinical studies, and self-initiated dropout rates are high in AN studies, making adequate recruitment difficult. In addition, full recovery often requires a long-term approach and multiple treatments. The result is a dearth of treatment studies for AN (Le Grange and Lock 2005).

Since the publication of the 2006 edition of the *Annual Review of Eating Disorders*, two randomized controlled trials (RCTs) of psychotherapy have been published (Lock *et al.* 2005; McIntosh *et al.* 2005). In terms of psychopharmacology studies, a multi-site study examining the efficacy of fluoxetine for relapse prevention represents the largest clinical drug trial to date for AN (Walsh *et al.* 2006). In addition, preliminary data have emerged on the potential efficacy of atypical antipsychotic medication for individuals with AN (Attia *et al.* 2005; Mondraty *et al.* 2005). Contributing to our understanding of the long-term efficacy of certain treatments, Lock *et al.* (2006a) reported one follow-up study for adolescents. In addition, Halmi *et al.* (2005) reported on the issues of treatment acceptability and completion, based on a study of 122 adults with AN. Thus, although only a limited number of treatment studies on AN were published during the last two years, they have a wide scope and contribute to the empirical knowledge base with regard to psychotherapy and medication interventions for both adolescents and adults with AN. In addition, several investigations that have examined the efficacy of family treatment for children with AN, therapeutic alliance and alternative treatment approaches have contributed to an emerging empirical foundation for treatment of AN.

Literature review

Family-based therapy for adolescents

Family therapy for younger patients with AN has been an essential component of treatment at the well-known Maudsley Hospital in London. Now known as the Maudsley method, this family-based treatment for AN was developed by Dare and Eisler (2000). More recently, Lock *et al.* (2001) further operationalized and empirically evaluated the efficacy of this approach for treating adolescents with AN. Two recent case series report on the feasibility and effectiveness of this manualized family-based therapy as a treatment option for adolescents and children with AN (Le Grange *et al.* 2005; Lock *et al.* 2006). In this series of case studies, Le Grange *et al.* (2005) reported that approximately 90% of their sample of 45 children and adolescents experienced full recovery or marked improvement over the course of treatment, with 56% gaining to more than 85% of ideal body weight (IBW) and resuming menses, and 33% achieving more than 85% of IBW without resuming normal menses.

Lock *et al.* (2006c) conducted a retrospective chart review to compare the pre- and post-treatment characteristics of children aged 12 years or younger ($n = 32$) who were treated with manualized family-based therapy with those of adolescents (aged 13 or older; $n = 78$) who received the same type of treatment. The majority of the children aged 12 years or younger (75%; $n = 24$) were seen in the context of routine clinical care at two university-based eating disorder treatment centers. The adolescents who constituted the comparison group in this report participated in a previous controlled clinical trial conducted by the same research group (Lock *et al.* 2005). The authors reported a treatment completion rate of 84.4% and a weight recovery rate of 96% for the case series of children. These findings were comparable to those reported for the adolescent comparison group, and provide preliminary support for the potential efficacy of family-based therapy for this younger age group.

In 2005, Lock and colleagues published the results of an RCT that compared short-term (up to 10 sessions over six months) with long-term (up to 20 sessions over 12 months) family-based treatment in 86 adolescents with AN. In total, 77 of the 86 participants (90%) completed treatment. It was found that 96% of the participants ended treatment with a body mass index (BMI) above 17.5 kg/m^2, and 67% had a BMI of 20 kg/m^2 or higher and a global Eating Disorder Examination (EDE) score within two standard deviations of normal at the end of the study. No statistically significant differences were detected between the treatment groups on any of the primary or secondary outcome measures, suggesting that six months of treatment may be as beneficial as a longer treatment for the resolution of AN symptoms in young patients with a relatively short duration of illness.

To compare the long-term outcomes of the adolescents who had received either a short-term or long-term course of family-based therapy in their original study, Lock *et al.* (2006a) conducted a follow-up study between two and six years after completion of the original trial (Lock *et al.* 2005). In total, 71 of the 86 original subjects (82.6%) participated in the follow-up assessment. The mean length of follow-up was four years, and the mean age of participants was 19.2 years at the time of follow-up. As reported above, these groups did not differ at the end of treatment, nor did they differ at follow-up on BMI, global EDE score, use of hospitalization for medical problems relating to AN, or further medical or psychological treatment since the end of the original study. Of the 71 follow-up participants, 63 (89%) weighed more than 90% of their ideal body weight. Although these findings are promising, a limitation of this follow-up study is that only 39.4% of the participants actually attended assessments in person, while information for the remaining participants was collected by telephone from the participant or a parent.

Utilizing the data set from the study by Lock *et al.* (2005), two secondary analyses were conducted in order to identify predictors of dropout and remission in the adolescent sample (Lock *et al.* 2006b) and examine the role of therapeutic alliance in predicting treatment outcome for the adolescents who were randomized to the 12-month family-based treatment (Pereira *et al.* 2006). In the first study, the presence of a comorbid disorder and longer-term treatment predicted a higher rate of dropout. In terms of symptom remission, comorbid psychiatric illness was associated with lower rates of remission. Higher age, more child behavior problems, and greater problems in family relationships were inversely correlated with remission.

In the study by Pereira *et al.* (2006), three researchers who were not involved in the original data collection assessed the quality of the therapeutic alliance between the therapist and adolescent and the therapist and parent during two full-length family therapy sessions using the Working Alliance Inventory–Observer (WAI-O). Separate ratings of therapeutic alliance were obtained for the adolescent and one of their parents early (about session six) and late (about session 16) in treatment. Overall, parents had higher ratings than adolescents on all early measures of therapeutic alliance. A strong early therapeutic alliance with parents predicted lower dropout, while a strong therapeutic alliance with parents later in treatment predicted greater adolescent weight gain at the end of treatment. Therapeutic alliance with adolescents did not predict overall weight change, but a strong early therapeutic alliance with adolescents was associated with weight gain early in treatment. Early weight gain in turn predicted overall decreases in EDE scores and total weight gain over the course of treatment. The authors concluded that therapeutic alliance with both adolescents and parents is important for facilitating a positive outcome in family-based therapy, as the former is correlated with weight gain and the latter with decreased likelihood of dropout.

Individual psychotherapy for adults

In many ways the study of therapeutic interventions for adults with AN presents a greater challenge for researchers than does the investigation of effective treatments for adolescents. Once an individual reaches maturity, her parents have less psychological and legal leverage in decision making regarding treatment, and many adults with AN have developed a chronic condition that is often associated with multiple treatments and relapses over the course of the illness. Thus documentation of evidence-based treatment for adult AN is limited, and there is a great need to expand our systematic examination of various treatment options for adults with AN, given the high morbidity and mortality associated with adult AN.

One recent clinical trial (McIntosh *et al.* 2005) randomized 56 women who met modified criteria for AN to receive 20 manual-based sessions of either cognitive–behavioral therapy (CBT), interpersonal psychotherapy (IPT) or non-specific supportive clinical management (NSCM) over a minimum period of 20 weeks. Each participant completed a battery of physical and psychological assessments at intake, after her tenth therapy session, and then again after her final session. The primary outcome variable was global AN rating, a scale developed specifically for this study.

At the end of the trial, 9% of the patients had a good outcome, 21% had improved considerably, and 70% did not complete treatment or showed little or no improvement. Contrary to the authors' a priori hypothesis, NSCM was found to be superior to IPT, while CBT did not differ significantly from either of the other two therapies. When considering the outcome of only the treatment completers (patients who attended at least 15 of the 20 therapy sessions), NSCM was superior to both CBT and IPT in terms of global AN rating, while no difference was found between the two more specialized psychotherapies. However, it is important to note that regardless of treatment condition, the majority of these individuals did not show considerable improvement, which suggests that all three of these treatments need to be enhanced or adapted further in order to achieve a better outcome.

The unexpected finding that NSCM was somewhat more effective than CBT and IPT in the study by McIntosh *et al.* (2005) led the investigators to publish an article describing the development, implementation and goals of this treatment, which was renamed 'specialist supportive clinical management' (SSCM) (McIntosh *et al.* 2006). In the SSCM treatment, therapists responded to the patient's presentation of issues for discussion, while still focusing on the resumption of normal eating (i.e. increasing the regularity, variety and quantity of food) with the aim of bringing about weight gain. This component of the SSCM treatment is also a core component of CBT, and thus it may be that the less structured components of SSCM were especially important to its increased acceptability and efficacy.

The description of treatments by McIntosh *et al.* (2006) raises important issues for the implementation of psychotherapy trials. Although the goal of 'meeting clients where they are' should be a priority in all treatments, many first-generation manuals for psychotherapy trials articulate a relatively fixed agenda and sequence of treatment, assuming a 'readiness to change' on the part of individuals. These manuals focus on aspects of attitudinal and behavioral change that may be more achievable once issues of engagement and motivation have been addressed more fully. In the study by McIntosh *et al.* (2006) it may be that the greater flexibility of approach contributed to its efficacy. Certainly engagement and motivation can be fully addressed from multiple theoretical perspectives, including CBT and IPT. In fact, fundamental to CBT is a collaborative approach in setting therapeutic goals with clients, ongoing and integrated cost–benefit evaluation of the disorder, and intentional, incremental exploration and experimentation with change. Similarly, in the initial phase of IPT, the focus of treatment is on identifying what is most salient and motivating for the client in terms of interpersonal relationships. Perhaps one of the most far-reaching implications of the study by McIntosh *et al.* (2006) is that it suggests the possibility that treatment manuals for psychotherapy trials need to provide greater flexibility in order to maximize these components of treatment so that the actual course of treatment is more fully tailored to address individualized needs (as would be the case in good clinical practice). It will be useful to evaluate whether therapeutic efficacy and treatment outcome are enhanced in subsequent generations of psychotherapy trials that utilize more flexible treatment manuals and that provide optional modules.

Psychotherapy studies for adults with AN are needed to replicate and extend the study conducted by McIntosh *et al.* (2006), given that this investigation had a relatively small sample size, a high drop-out rate, and the analyses were largely based on treatment completers. It will be important for future research to explore further the issues of treatment retention, manual-based treatment components and enhanced flexibility to develop enhanced evidence-based psychotherapy interventions for adults with AN.

Pharmacological interventions

Over the past two years, only one randomized multi-site trial has examined the efficacy of pharmacological treatments for adults with AN (Walsh *et al.* 2006). This study sought to determine whether fluoxetine was more effective than placebo in promoting psychological and behavioral recovery and prolonging time to relapse in patients with AN immediately following weight restoration. A total of 93 women who met the DSM-IV criteria for AN (with the exception of the amenorrhea criterion) received a course of intensive inpatient or day-program treatment until they had reached and maintained a BMI of at least 19 kg/m^2 for two weeks, at which time they were randomized to receive either fluoxetine or placebo together with outpatient CBT. Medication was initiated one week prior to discharge, and the dosage was increased from 20 mg/day to 60 mg/day over a one-week period. This dosage was maintained throughout the trial unless there were adverse effects or clinical deterioration (at which time the dose was decreased or increased, respectively). All of the participants were treated for up to 12 months with a combination of medication and a form of manual-based CBT that has been found to be useful in reducing relapse in AN (Pike *et al.* 2003). Every four weeks the participants completed a battery of psychological assessments that evaluated disturbed eating behaviors and cognitions, depression, anxiety and self-esteem. They also completed measures of obsessionality and quality of life before randomization, after six months of treatment, and at termination of the study.

The primary outcome measure was time to relapse. Relapse was defined as maintaining a BMI at or below 16.5 kg/m^2 for two consecutive weeks, experiencing severe medical complications as a result of the eating disorder, being at imminent risk for suicide, or developing another severe psychiatric disorder that required treatment. Secondary analyses examined group differences in symptoms over time using random-effects regression models. The fluoxetine and placebo groups did not differ significantly with regard to the percentages of patients who completed the study or the average number of psychotherapy sessions. In addition, the groups did not differ with regard to time to relapse. In secondary analyses, the Beck Anxiety Inventory was the only measure on which the groups differed significantly. Specifically, individuals in the fluoxetine group reported a greater reduction in anxiety than those in the placebo group. Overall, the study produced no convincing evidence that fluoxetine provided significant benefit compared with placebo, as time to relapse, rate of study completion, BMI, and clinical measures at termination of the study were comparable across the groups.

Olanzapine is an atypical antipsychotic medication with a known side-effect of weight gain. Recent investigations have explored its potential application in the treatment of AN. Case reports and uncontrolled data suggest that olanzapine may be helpful in patients with AN (Powers *et al.* 2002; Barbarich *et al.* 2004). Mondraty *et al.* (2005) conducted a controlled trial of 15 inpatients with AN who were randomized to receive either olanzapine or chlorpromazine for the duration of their hospital stay. The study found that patients in both groups gained a similar amount of weight, but that those who received olanzapine experienced less ruminative thinking. The study was limited by its small size, the fact that the study treatment was adjunctive to inpatient treatment, and the somewhat discrepant doses used in the trial (the mean dose of olanzapine was 10 mg, whereas a relatively lower dose of 50 mg of chlorpromazine was used).

Attia *et al.* (2005) reported results from a randomized controlled pilot study that compared olanzapine with aripiprazole in 22 patients with AN. The study aimed to assess the feasibility, acceptability and general effectiveness of atypical antipsychotic agents in this clinical population, and to describe any differences in response to these medications. Like olanzapine, aripiprazole is an atypical antipsychotic medication, but in contrast to olanzapine it does not have the same side-effect of weight gain. Patients who received olanzapine showed a mean weight gain of 2.2 lbs $\pm$ 6.3 lbs, compared with a mean weight loss of -1.2 $\pm$ 5.1 lbs for the group that received aripiprazole, representing a statistically significant difference in total weekly weight change. In addition, anxiety scores improved in patients who received olanzapine but not in those who received aripiprazole. The mean dose achieved was 4.4 $\pm$ 3.2 mg olanzapine and 8.1 $\pm$ 5.9 mg aripiprazole. The study was notable for the great difficulty in recruiting the study sample. In addition, the rate of patient-initiated drop-out was high, with 17 of 22 randomized patients not completing the full 12 weeks of the medication trial. These practical considerations suggest that the viability of this treatment may be limited to a small subset of individuals with AN.

Treatment acceptability and compliance

Treatment acceptability and compliance is an important issue across all clinical care. However, as noted above, it is particularly complicated and challenging in the treatment of AN because ambivalence about treatment is the norm and medical factors often require withdrawal from treatment. In a study of 122 individuals with AN, Halmi *et al.* (2005) examined treatment acceptability and completion for CBT, fluoxetine, and combined CBT and fluoxetine. Of the 122 randomized patients, 21 (17%) were withdrawn from the study for medical reasons, and 56 of the remaining 101 patients (55%) dropped out of treatment for a variety of reasons. In total, 89 of the 122 patients (73%) accepted the treatment to which they were randomized (defined as staying in treatment for at least five weeks). Patients who were randomized to receive medication without CBT accepted treatment at a significantly lower rate than those who were randomized to receive CBT or combination treatment (56% and 81% rate of acceptance, respectively). The treatment completion rate was 27% for patients who were randomized to receive medication alone, 43% for those who received CBT alone, and 38% for the combination group.

Summary of important findings and clinical implications

Overall, the most promising lines of research into treatments for AN have been in the area of psychotherapeutic interventions. Manualized family-based treatment has consistently led to substantial symptom reduction in the children and adolescents who have been treated with this form of therapy. Results from two studies published in 2005 and 2006 (Lock *et al.* 2005, 2006a) provide promising evidence for this treatment approach for young and relatively recent onset cases of AN. However, it is important to note that the Maudsley family treatment has not been compared with alternative treatments in rigorous RCTs. Therefore the encouraging results may not be specific to this treatment, but may be largely a function of the fact that this group is developmentally young and that the onset of AN is relatively recent. It is essential that future studies assess the specific efficacy of family treatment as compared with other interventions.

Compared with the adolescent literature, results from psychotherapy research in adults (McIntosh *et al.* 2005) show less efficacy for outpatient treatments with regard to weight restoration, with 70% of participants either terminating treatment prematurely or gaining little or no benefit from treatment. In contrast, evidence is emerging to support the role of outpatient CBT in preventing relapse among weight-restored individuals (Pike *et al.* 2003). However, the study and follow-up publication by McIntosh *et al.* (2005, 2006) provide helpful information concerning what may be the useful ingredients for an effective form of psychotherapy for the treatment of adults with AN. Clearly, future research into these and other psychotherapeutic interventions for AN is warranted.

In the area of pharmacological treatments for AN, we still lack any compelling evidence for a medication intervention that would be widely acceptable and efficacious. The largest extant RCT on treatment for AN, conducted by Walsh *et al.* (2006), offers no support for fluoxetine, and the smaller studies by Mondraty *et al.* (2005) and Attia *et al.* (2005) offer some evidence of efficacy for certain antipsychotic medications, but low acceptability from patients' perspectives. Again, other avenues of pharmacological treatment need to be explored in future clinical trials.

Future directions

Psychotherapy studies

A multi-site trial of the Maudsley method is currently under way to further investigate the efficacy of family therapy in AN treatment (CRISP 2007). In addition, Zucker *et al.* (2006) reported another promising treatment approach for adolescents with eating disorders using a Group Parent Training Program (GPT). A total of 16 families of adolescents diagnosed with AN, bulimia nervosa or eating disorder not otherwise specified participated in approximately 16 sessions of GPT and then completed the Consumer Satisfaction/Treatment

Effectiveness Survey (CSTE), which rated their level of satisfaction with specific aspects of the program. Overall, the evaluation of GPT was positive, with 100% of participants reporting mild or strong agreement with statements such as "I would recommend this group to other parents" and "The parent training group was essential for the improvement of my child." Evidence from this study supports the acceptability of GPT as a novel approach to the management of adolescents with eating disorders. However, its efficacy in terms of ameliorating the eating disorders has yet to be determined. A clinical trial is currently in progress to gather more information on the effectiveness of GPT (CRISP 2007).

With regard to long-term recovery following weight restoration, the promising data for CBT documented by Pike et al. (2003) need to be replicated with a larger sample. The potentially long-term course of AN and the frequent relapses reported by individuals who achieve weight restoration but fail to maintain it suggest that this phase of treatment is critical to lasting recovery. The current trend is to shorten hospital stays, and this is associated with more frequent relapse and rehospitalization (Willer et al. 2005). Thus, the development of effective treatments for this stage of care is especially important. In particular, for individuals who have had AN for more than a relatively short duration, enhanced or alternative psychotherapy interventions need to be developed to further facilitate lasting recovery.

Medication trials

Despite a long history of medication trials for AN, and despite the widely recognized biological factors intrinsic to AN, to date no psychopharmacological interventions have been found to be consistently effective. It is important to continue to explore alternative classes of medication and novel medications in the hope that they may eventually lead to important contributions to the clinical care of individuals with AN.

Improving our methods

Future studies of AN need to be conducted collaboratively across multiple sites in order to increase sample sizes and accelerate data collection. In addition, standardized measures and criteria for assessing and describing outcome are essential. Depending on how we measure outcome and how we define recovery, the same individuals may be described as achieving poor, partial or full states of recovery (Courturier and Lock 2006). In turn, different treatments earn the reputation of being extremely effective or ineffective at least in part as a function of how outcome is specified.

New treatment settings for AN patient care, such as residential treatments, are rapidly developing. Although these may be positive developments, given the high costs associated with hospital inpatient care and the limitations of hospital-based programs, these residential programs are also expensive, and their efficacy is largely unknown. According to a recent study (Frisch et al. 2006), the average length of stay in residential treatment settings in the USA is 83 days, at an average cost of almost $1000/day. Given that residential treatment programs for eating disorders are extremely heterogeneous and largely un-regulated, further research is necessary to determine the effectiveness of such programs.

AN research could benefit from closer examination of predictors and me-diators of treatment effects to determine whether there are subsets of patients who respond to particular interventions and whether there are interactions between different factors that account for treatment effects. For example, Mayer et al. (2007) found that body composition – specifically the percentage of body fat – predicted outcome among weight-restored patients with AN participating in an outpatient, relapse-prevention treatment. Higher percentage body fat predicted a rating of fair, good or full recovery on the Morgan–Russell scale in patients who received CBT for one year as part of the previously mentioned fluoxetine versus placebo relapse prevention trial (Walsh et al. 2006). Given the dramatic biological components of AN, increasing our understanding of the biological processes associated with different stages of the disorder, and utilizing these data to inform treatment interventions, is another area that could expand greatly in the future. Recent data on basal metabolic rate (BMR) (Forman-Hoffnam et al. 2006) suggest that individuals with AN experience a significant increase in BMR during nutritional rehabilitation on an inpatient unit, but BMR returns to expected values within three weeks of commencement of treatment. Such data could usefully be applied to nutritional planning for AN patients during the early stages of weight gain.

Conclusion

Treatment for AN is slowly building an empirical foundation, and a number of important studies have been published in the last two years that contribute to our knowledge of medication and psychotherapy interventions for adults, adolescents and children. However, major challenges in AN treatment research include the relatively low prevalence rate of the disorder, ambivalence about treatment and recovery, and significant medical complications that require frequent adaptations of treatment. Future investigations need to recruit large samples in order to advance our understanding of treatment efficacy, and they need to focus on enhancing treatment acceptability and completion to improve retention rates, so that a more definitive understanding of treatment efficacy can be achieved.

References

(References included from the targeted review years are preceded by one asterisk. References preceded by three asterisks are of particular significance. The significance is explained by a short commentary following the complete reference.)

Agras WS, Brandt HA, Bulik CM, Dolan-Sewell R, Fairburn CG, Halmi KA *et al.* (2004) Report of the National Institutes of Health workshop on overcoming barriers to treatment research in anorexia nervosa. *International Journal of Eating Disorders,* **35:** 509–21.

*Attia E, Kaplan AS, Schroeder L, Federici A and Staab R (2005) *Atypical antipsychotic medication in anorexia nervosa.* Eating Disorders Research Society Annual Meeting, Toronto, Canada, 29 September 2005.

Barbarich NC, McConaha CW, Gaskill J, La Via M, Frank GK, Achenbach S *et al.* (2004) An open trial of olanzapine in anorexia nervosa. *Journal of Clinical Psychiatry,* **65:** 1480–2.

***Couturier J and Lock J (2006) What is recovery in adolescent anorexia nervosa? *International Journal of Eating Disorders,* **39:** 550–55.

The field lacks standardized outcome assessment for AN. This study illustrates the impact that different operational definitions of recovery have on a single data set. Depending on the criteria employed, the same individuals may be classified as having a poor, intermediate or good outcome. Given that standards for outcome assessment are lacking, the development of a coherent database on treatment efficacy is dramatically hampered. The authors of this study offer recommendations for standardizing outcome assessment.

CRISP (Computer Retrieval of Information on Scientific Projects) Hit List (2007); http://crisp.cit.nih.gov/crisp/crisp_lib.query.

Dare C and Eisler I (2000) A multi-family group day treatment programme for adolescent eating disorders. *European Eating Disorders Review,* **8:** 4–18.

*Forman-Hoffnam VL, Ruffin T and Schultz SK (2006) Basal metabolic rate in anorexia nervosa patients: using appropriate predictive equations during the refeeding process. *Annals of Clinical Psychiatry,* **18:** 123–7.

*Frisch MJ, Herzog DB and Franko DL (2006) Residential treatment for eating disorders. *International Journal of Eating Disorders,* **39:** 434–42.

*Halmi KA, Agras WS, Crow S, Mitchell J, Wilson GT, Bryson SW *et al.* (2005) Predictors of treatment acceptance and completion in anorexia nervosa. *Archives of General Psychiatry,* **62:** 776–81.

*Le Grange D and Lock J (2005) The dearth of psychological treatment studies for anorexia nervosa. *International Journal of Eating Disorders,* **37:** 79–91.

*Le Grange D, Binford R and Loeb KL (2005) Manualized family-based treatment for anorexia nervosa: a case series. *Journal of the American Academy of Child and Adolescent Psychiatry,* **44:** 41–6.

Lock J, le Grange D, Agras WS and Dare C (2001) *Treatment Manual for Anorexia Nervosa: a family-based approach.* New York: Guilford Press.

***Lock J, Agras WS, Bryson S and Kraemer HC (2005) A comparison of short- and long-term family therapy for adolescent anorexia nervosa. *Journal of the American Academy of Child and Adolescent Psychiatry,* **44:** 632–9.

This paper provides empirical evidence for the Maudsley model of family therapy. Although several clinical descriptions of this treatment approach pre-date this publication, this is the first randomized clinical trial that documents its clinical efficacy. The results of the trial suggest that this is a promising approach for

adolescents with relatively short duration of AN. However, it should be noted that the comparison focuses on intensity and duration of treatment, and does not compare the Maudsley approach with alternative therapies.

*Lock J, Couturier J and Agras WS (2006a) Comparison of long-term outcomes in adolescents with anorexia nervosa treatment with family therapy. *Journal of the American Academy of Child and Adolescent Psychiatry*, **45**: 666–72.

*Lock J, Couturier J, Bryson S and Agras S (2006b) Predictors of dropout and remission in family therapy for adolescent anorexia nervosa in a randomized clinical trial. *International Journal of Eating Disorders*, **39**: 639–47.

*Lock J, le Grange D, Forsberg S and Hewell K (2006c) Is family therapy useful for treating children with anorexia nervosa? Results of a case series. *Journal of the American Academy of Child and Adolescent Psychiatry*, **45**: 1323–8.

***McIntosh VVW, Jordan J, Carter FA, Luty SE, McKenzie JM, Bulik CM *et al.* (2005) Three psychotherapies for anorexia nervosa: a randomized, controlled trial. *American Journal of Psychiatry*, **162**: 741–7.

This study provides important data on the efficacy of three outpatient psychotherapies for adult AN, and it reports provocative findings with regard to treatment outcome. However, the study will need to be replicated before conclusions can be drawn with regard to any of these treatments, given the limitations due to the small sample size and high drop-out rate.

*McIntosh VVW, Jordan J, Luty SE, Carter FA, McKenzie JM, Bulik CM *et al.* (2006) Specialist supportive clinical management for anorexia nervosa. *International Journal of Eating Disorders*, **39**: 625–32.

*Mayer L, Roberto CA, Glasofer DR, Etu SF, Gallagher D, Wang J *et al.* (2007) Percent body fat predicts outcome in anorexia nervosa. *American Journal of Psychiatry*, **164**: 970–2.

*Mondraty N, Birmingham CL, Touyz S, Sundakov V, Chapman L and Beumont P (2005) Randomized controlled trial of olanzapine in the treatment of cognitions in anorexia nervosa. *Australasian Psychiatry*, **13**: 72–5.

Morgan HG and Hayward AE (1988) Clinical assessment of anorexia nervosa. The Morgan-Russell outcome assessment schedule. *British Journal of Psychiatry*, **152**: 367–71.

Pereira T, Lock J and Oggins J (2006) Role of therapeutic alliance in family therapy for adolescent anorexia nervosa. *International Journal of Eating Disorders*, **39**: 677–83.

Pike KM, Walsh BT, Vitousek K, Wilson GT and Bauer J (2003) Cognitive behavioral therapy in the post-hospitalization treatment of anorexia nervosa. *American Journal of Psychiatry*, **160**: 2046–9.

Powers PS, Santana CA and Bannon YS (2002) Olanzapine in the treatment of anorexia nervosa: an open label trial. *International Journal of Eating Disorders*, **32**: 146–54.

***Walsh BT, Kaplan AS, Attia E, Olmsted M, Parides M, Carter JC *et al.* (2006) Fluoxetine after weight restoration in anorexia nervosa: a randomized controlled trial. *Journal of the American Medical Association*, **295**: 2605–12.

This is the largest extant randomized controlled trial of treatment of AN. Although earlier studies offered preliminary support for fluoxetine after weight restoration in AN treatment, the results from this multi-site study indicate that when delivered in conjunction with CBT, there is no evidence that fluoxetine is of any benefit at this stage of AN treatment.

*Willer MG, Thuras P and Crow SJ (2005) Implications of the changing use of hospitalization to treat anorexia nervosa. *American Journal of Psychiatry*, **162**: 2374–6.

*Zucker NL, Marcus M and Bulik C (2006) A group parent-training program: a novel approach for eating disorder management. *Eating and Weight Disorders*, **11**: 78–82.

Index